REAL MEN DON'T GO WOKE

REAL MEN DON'T GO WOKE

The Book They Would Not Publish.
The Truth That Must Be Told.

DR. GILDA CARLE

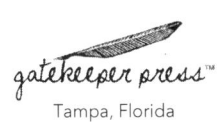

Tampa, Florida

The content associated with this book is the sole work and responsibility of the author. Gatekeeper Press had no involvement in the generation of this content.

Real Men Don't Go Woke

Published by Gatekeeper Press
7853 Gunn Hwy., Suite 209
Tampa, FL 33626
www.GatekeeperPress.com

Copyright © 2024 by Dr. Gilda Carle
All rights reserved. Neither this book, nor any parts within it may be sold or reproduced in any form or by any electronic or mechanical means, including information storage and retrieval systems, without permission in writing from the author. The only exception is by a reviewer, who may quote short excerpts in a review.

The cover design, interior formatting, typesetting, and editorial work for this book are entirely the product of the author. Gatekeeper Press did not participate in and is not responsible for any aspect of these elements.

Library of Congress Control Number:

ISBN (hardcover): 9781662957253
ISBN (paperback): 9781662957260
eISBN: 9781662957277

DEDICATION

For all men
and the women who love them.

INSIDE THE PUBLISHING SAGA

The first book I wrote got a million dollar advance because of my celebrity status on national TV. I have since written 19 books. I've also been a columnist for The Today Show, Match.com, The National Enquirer, and countless popular magazines and newspapers. I have been a relationship expert on Dateline, Howard Stern, Sally Jessy Raphael, and most national talk and news shows, culminating in Twentieth Century Fox producing a TV pilot for "The Dr. Gilda Show." I have also been teaching graduate MBA students for decades. That's my background of knowledge, accomplishment, and success as an educator.

However, after submitting this book to a literary agent, I was told the big five book publishers will not publish anti-woke books. The agent explained that the female decision-making 30-something editors were woke, and they use the clout of their positions to block and cancel any premise that does not resonate with theirs.

The leanings of the 30-something editors the agent described were in keeping with the research cited in this book: Women of that age group subscribe to woke doctrines, while their male counterparts are moving toward conservativism. Experts note how this political gender divide is ruining the potential for mental health and sound relationships especially among Gen Zs and millennials. Ironically, unhappy woke singles of all ages are among those who seek my counsel as a relationship expert when they strike out at love.

Older men are also confused by this sudden woke culture, and so they go along to get along instead of standing up for what they believe. Any kind of lying—even to oneself—tears a soul apart—and too many men today are sick and suffering. But trying to keep peace makes sense because in this culture, disagreeing could get a guy cancelled, sued, ostracized, blocked, or fired.

I was driven to write this book because of the pain punctuating so many men's lives. It originally had a different title. But the agent's words registered: *Wokesters will cancel my book before they even see it!*

So, I did what any self-respecting, grounded, literate woman would do: I boldly changed the title to include the word "woke," and reclaimed control of the dissemination of my important research.

FOREWORD

Men are an endangered species. Male suicides are four times higher than those of women, making male suicide a public health emergency. Non-Hispanic American Indian and Alaskan Native men top the list, followed by non-Hispanic white men.

Men's rights expert and author Warren Farrell warns of "The Boy Crisis," the name of his 6-part lecture series at Peterson Academy, which I attended. He points to the frightening statistics in the U.S.: Boys aged 10 to 14 commit suicide at twice the rate of girls; boys 15 to 19 commit suicide four times the rate of girls; boys 20 to 24 commit suicide five to five-and-a-half times the rate of girls. These horrifying trends are also seen around the world throughout Europe, China, Japan, Sweden, and India.

Moreover, male life expectancy is steadily decreasing. Before COVID, male life expectancy went down 3 years in a row, a historical first, while female life expectancy remained the same.

Further, 90 percent of people who die at work are men.

Traditional masculinity boasts self-reliance, stoicism, strength, and toughness. Studies show how these traits can lead to emotional constriction, substance abuse, depression, aggression, and violence. Many men won't seek mental health support for their loneliness, depression, confusion, and anxiety for fear of seeming weak. Other men don't respect weakness, and women tend to prefer alphas. When a man does not meet the culture's expectations, his stress becomes monumental, and dysfunction and trauma set in.

Developmental psychologist Gary Barker studies men and boys worldwide as CEO and co-founder of the Equimundo Center for Masculinities and Social Justice. He cites that the version of manhood for most of the world today consists of outperforming others at all costs, not asking for help, not seeming vulnerable, using sex for conquest instead of intimacy and connection, demonstrating toughness, and applying violence to grab whatever is desired. He concludes, "We are literally dying of manhood."

Boys grow into men, so our culture should be mindful of how we treat male children. Farrell attributes "The Boy Crisis" to five causes:

1. dad-deprived boys
2. the belief for a half century that girls and women are powerless while male toxicity, male privilege, and male power rule

3. the void of purpose
4. the fear of attachment to someone they may lose
5. the culture repulsed by males who complain

Farrell admits, "I would not be hired at any university in the United States. That's how dangerous talking this way is." Jordan Peterson would rather that men seem dangerous than weak, as long as their sword is kept sheathed. The woke mindset would question why there's a need for a sword.

Maleness is in turmoil. So, it makes sense that a sector of the population is pushing the pendulum in the opposite direction from tradition. The new culture of wokeness is purported to rescue the imperfect male paradigm, as though the opposite gender has perfection nailed.

But there's pushback by men to return to what used to be. On a podcast with Bari Weiss, the founder and editor of The Free Press, Jerry Seinfeld inadvertently supported this book's title by saying, "I like a Real Man." He explained, "I miss dominant masculinity. Yeah, I get the toxic, but still, I like a Real Man." *Thank you for the plug, Jerry!*

Comedian Greg Gutfeld on his show on Fox News Channel agreed with Seinfeld's lament for a "dominant masculinity." Gutfeld said he misses the "bygone era of real men": "I miss the days when men were men and women were not." Kevin O'Leary, or Mr. Wonderful from Shark Tank, chided, "I'm pretty sure talking about what makes a manly man is racist."

Mixed race actor and former pro wrestler Tyrus supported alpha men with "We're good." These guys humorously swung at the new breed of woke masculinity consuming the media. Bill Maher's book, "What the Comedian Said Will Shock You," described that men have become wimps. "It's the result of having it drilled into us in recent years that masculinity is toxic and scary and unevolved."

According to the Urban Dictionary, the opposite of a Real Man is a "woke" or "socially submissive" man. Originating as slang among Black Americans, woke's popularity swelled in 2014 as part of the rhetoric of Black Lives Matter. Now, it has morphed to describe *men's abandonment of manhood*. When Black men are said to abandon their "blackness," they are derided as "Oreos." But when all men are asked to surrender their manhood, if they concur, they become what I call "Cheerios": Their outside may look solid, but their inside is empty. The abandonment of manhood is a death sentence for what boys are being trained to become. And it's problematic for men who can't be too weak or too strong, because both extremes label them as inadequate.

My research on this topic has spanned historical profiles, online conversations, real emails between men and women, news articles, documentaries, pop culture pieces, podcasts, online dating sites, audios, interviews, discussions with both genders, books, TV and radio shows, current events, conferences, lectures, and movies. Besides these sources, I am a divorced heterosexual female who dates heterosexual males, so I occupy a front-row seat to a vast array of dysfunctional behaviors.

Every character I exemplify in this book is based on a real person or situation. Some are laughable, and some are pitiful. But I find that men today are caught in a muddle of mystification about where they fit between woke and toxic. Celebrities' names are familiar, but civilian names, credentials, professions, ages, and locations have been altered to safeguard anonymity. Some of my examples are even composites of several people. But the behaviors are recognizable because they're omnipresent.

I wrote this book to support Real Men during these confusing times. "Woke" is today's buzzword. But this book also underscores that the opposite extreme of toxic masculinity does not define a Real Man, either. Developmental psychologist Niobe Way says that our culture has "gendered" what is fundamentally human. Like "thinking," "stoicism," "hardness," and "disconnection" are *supposed to be* masculine, and "feelings," "vulnerability," "softness," and "connection" are *supposed to be* feminine.

Heaven help a guy who steps out of his masculine lane! I once told a macho army fighter that I loved seeing his vulnerable side. After not understanding how vulnerability could be complimentary, he became insulted! Yet, Generation Woke pushes men to lose the masculine in order to also lose their alleged "toxicity." Men are perplexed on how to proceed.

"Real Men Don't Go Woke" takes traditional *supposed-to-be's* with which men are familiar and *adds* the other side of masculinity that has been suppressed, the side that drives men to suicide, murder/suicide, drugs, alcohol, porn abuse, job and career terminations, fractured relationships, and other dropout behaviors described here. This book upholds empowerment, self-worth, health, and longevity.

My five objectives are:

- #1: to explore heterosexual men's lives today: how they cope, how they hide, how they sabotage their emotional and physical health, and the dangerous outcomes of their loneliness. We are in the midst of a crisis!

- #2: to support healthy connections, behaviors, and lifestyles between hetero men and women.

- #3: to expose men's interpersonal problems because once something is mentionable, it is manageable—and we are all capable managers of our lives if only we have the tools.

- #4: to fill the expertise void left by the TV talk shows on which I spent years appearing. People were then able to tap expert advice to cope with interpersonal and mental health issues. That space is sorely missing today.

- #5: purely selfish: Strong heterosexual males make strong heterosexual partners for me and the daughters, granddaughters, and nieces who line up behind me. Women want men who proudly and honestly stand with a sturdy backbone and who transparently express their voices.

A man has only one escape from his old self, and that is to see a different self in the mirror of some woman's eyes.

—Clare Boothe Luce,
"The Women—It's All About Men," 1937

Luce's statement is important because most of the experts on boys and men offer perspectives through Tarzan's eyes. Jane's eyes provide a unique view. This book puts forth a mirror to reflect a different self of a strong *yet humanly vulnerable* man who expresses his truth without fear. That man will live a happier and healthier life.

—Dr. Gilda

PREFACE

I began my career as a teacher in the dangerous South Bronx. While I taught the kids language arts skills, they taught me street smarts. Their world was violent, and these street urchins knew how to manipulate and con their way into and around danger. Some survived, and some succumbed to gang warfare and drugs. There was always fighting.

When I started my Ph.D. at New York University, I became a student of the 4th Century BC Chinese general, military strategist, and philosopher Sun Tzu and his well-known tome, "The Art of War." If I could have returned to the South Bronx, could I have convinced my savvy street students to subdue an enemy without fighting? Since I never got that chance, I took my new knowledge to corporate America. I regularly consulted with, coached, and media trained executives from Wall Street to Main Street to communicate in ways to raise their bottom line.

Sun Tzu's writings taught me to observe current conditions, strategize moves that outsmart, and thrive in each interaction without warfare. Executives had never been exposed to principles that underscored that the true objective of war is *peace*. This philosophy embraces brain power over the banality of brawn. It requires deliberate strategic planning that cannot survive with a wishy-washy woke mindset. Assertive strength is the only position to take.

> *I hope you experience a love that inspires dancing instead of walking on eggshells.*
>
> —Thema Bryant,
> Psychologist, Minister, and Sacred Artist

Then national TV discovered me. Spending just two years on that medium led Twentieth Century Fox to produce a TV pilot for "The Dr. Gilda Show."

The South Bronx was the source of my moxie. (Incidentally, the school at which I taught was only a few blocks from Judge Judy's Bronx County Courthouse. Not even being aware of this fact, my TV audiences nicknamed me "the Judge Judy of Relationships.") Sun Tzu taught me to strategize each move. The combination of South Bronx spunk and business strategy proved to be a winning recipe for my success. I apply this formula in "Real Men Don't Go Woke."

CONTENTS

INTRODUCTION:
Woke Created a Wake

Part I:
MEN'S NEW FEELINGS

Chapter 1: Wounded 21

Chapter 2: Banished 25

Chapter 3: Shamed 39

Chapter 4: Unneeded 51

Chapter 5: Angry 57

Part II:
NEW WORLD CONDITIONING

Chapter 6: Masculinity's Numerical Score 69

Chapter 7: Softness is for Sissies 83

Chapter 8: But Macho Has a Price 87

Part III:
10 WAYS HETERO MEN HIDE

Chapter 9: Sex-Possessed 111

Chapter 10: Gender Bender 115

Chapter 11: Human Dropout 129

Chapter 12: Opportunist 135

Chapter 13: Credentials Extender 143

Chapter 14: Forked Tongue Wordsmith 147

Chapter 15: Cradle Robber 151

Chapter 16: Ghost 161

Chapter 17: Comatose Shutdown 177

Chapter 18: Long Distance Sprinter 189

Part IV:
SOLUTIONS FOR EMOTIONAL DETOX

Chapter 19: Toxic Men in Trouble 199

Chapter 20: Why Do Good Men Stay Silent? 207

Chapter 21: Check Your Emotional History 211

Chapter 22: Simple Steps to Reconstruct a Spine 215

Part V:
REAL MEN WHO STAND UP

Chapter 23: Chris Rock 227
  Responds to The Slap—One Year Later............................... 227

Chapter 24: Saifullah Khan 229
  Sues to Reclaim Life after Rape Acquittal.......................... 229

Chapter 25: Sylvester Stallone..231
  Refuses Bud Light's $100 Million Endorsement Deal 231

Chapter 26: Greg O'Brien...233
  Videos His Demeaning Fight against Alzheimer's 233

Chapter 27: Johnny Depp...235
  Defeats Ex-Wife in Defamation Suit 235

Chapter 28: Dr. Peter McCullough...239
  World Expert on COVID Opposes
  Government Mandates.. 239

Chapter 29: Bill Ackman 243
  Shouts What Others Only Whisper: "DEI Is Racist" 243

Chapter 30: Ted Sarandos...251
  Defends Netflix's Programming No Matter
  Who Is Offended... 251

Chapter 31: Dan Crenshaw 253
   Blinded Former Navy Seal Touts
   "Never Be a Victim".. 253

Chapter 32: Ricky Gervais..255
   Pushes the Oscar Envelope of Controversy....................... 255

Chapter 33: Dr. Jordan Peterson..259
   Leads the Way for Strong Men, Loses License
   and University Credentials... 259

Chapter 34: Kevin Sorbo 265
   Exits Hollywood's Woke Agenda that Mocks Men 265

Chapter 35: Jon Stewart 267
   Quits Apple TV Show when He's Refused
   Creative Control 267

Chapter 36: Unknown Man 271
   Confronts Abusive Ex and Kids—
   to Internet Applause!... 271

Chapter 37: YOU 275
   If You Haven't Yet Claimed Your Voice,
   the Time is Now!.. 275

CONCLUSION:
Every Setback Re-Sets Us for a Better Path

SOURCES FOR EXPANSION 283

INTRODUCTION

Woke Created a Wake

As a relationship expert during this woke age, women continue to ask me where the Real Men are. It's true that "woke" does not exactly conjure up a manly "gladiator." But disenchantment with the male persona is nothing new. Issues questioning lost masculinity dated back to 1835 when Washington Irving criticized wealthy Americans for sending their boys to Europe to become "effeminate." He urged young men to pump up their "manliness" by working on the prairies. Over a century later, Arthur Schlesinger, Jr. wrote a 1958 essay in Esquire magazine that the American male had lost his toughness.

Now the question is how "masculine" masculinity should be regarding today's woke standards.

Reacting to a joke that excoriated him, Elon Musk shot back, "It is rather tragic to see an otherwise capable comedian like John Oliver become weak sauce. The reason he is not very funny these days is because he is too keen to pander to wokeness," thereby solidifying "wokeness" as the new curse word. Oliver retaliated by asking, "WTF's he talking about?" Oliver described Musk as thin-skinned and weak himself. This back-and-forth doesn't just depict two well-known men arguing about the extremes of masculinity during these times; it represents a genuine divide in how men enact their masculine roles.

Years ago, the corporate consulting company I created trained executives in the "soft," non-technical skills that were often the most difficult to grasp. Soft skill leadership includes problem-solving, teamwork, conflict management, listening, creativity, adaptability, critical thinking, and decision-making, all of whose requirements change according to the needs of the audience and the circumstances. Adept soft skills include thinking on your feet or your seat and acting quickly. I was routinely in Fortune 500 corporations, designing training programs for leaders. Even back then, soft skills were not deemed "manly" and were probably more attributable to females whose numbers had not yet begun to surge in the workforce. Therefore, the men in my programs were often resistant to mastering these proficiencies.

But the world was changing. By 2020, a TD Ameritrade survey found that 50 percent of women outearned or made the same income as their spouses, a huge leap from fewer than 4 percent of women in 1960. Therefore, the male "provider" model began to disappear. Many men felt ashamed for not living up to their fathers' role modeling.

Author Brene Brown says, "Men's shame usually displays as being pissed off." The pissed-offness of men today takes many forms, depending on the culture.

In Italy, the custom is for men in their thirties and forties to continue to live with Mama. As in the United States, Italy humiliates them as "Mama's boys." But as more mamas preserve their good looks and healthy bodies, they want to have a life for themselves after their kids are grown. One 75-year-old Italian mother, separated from her two sons' father and living off her pension, had had enough freeloading by her progeny. Whatever money she had went to the upkeep of the home and food for her "parasite" sons (as she called them), aged 40 and 42. As adult males, the sons were fully employed, continued to live with Mama rent-free, and refused to take responsibility for the house or do chores. So, Mama Mia filed a lawsuit with the courts to evict them.

The judge called the sons "big babies" and said, "There is no provision in the legislation which attributes to the adult child the unconditional right to remain in the home exclusively owned by the parents." So, Mama won. But, without shame, both grown sons lawyered up and countersued Mama to stop her from evicting them! This situation occurred in 2023, and these grown men in their 40s just couldn't get themselves to accept responsibility. The Italian judge responded that the sons could no longer expect their parents to uphold the maintenance obligation once they reached a certain age.

Coincidentally, about 20 years ago, I met a hip divorced

Italian American mother in her early 60s. She babied her adult son of 36, not unlike Italian mothers worldwide. She cooked for him, did his laundry, and provided a spotless house while he went to school, became a licensed exterminator, and began making a good living as an entrepreneur. Yet he still wanted to live with my friend. Mom had an active social life. She felt that needing to feel responsible for him was holding her back from living again. Despite her gentle cajoling, the woman couldn't get rid of the son she spoiled.

Finally fed up, one day, when he was at work, she packed her son's bags and left them on the front steps of her house. When he returned home that evening, she told him to follow her car in his truck. She drove to the local YMCA, where she announced he would lodge. He was shocked! He argued that this never happened in their long familial line of Italians. He complained that his mom hadn't even put him in a hotel. A few days later, the freeloader found his own apartment—and his way in the world. Nobody could believe such an overprotective and nurturing Italian mother would take such drastic action. But it worked. A few years later, he got married and raised a family. Then, he thanked his mom for finally pushing him to grow up!

Many woke young men live rent-free in their parents' basements with no goal of independence. What is this doing to that generation, other than raising malcontented kids who complain and rally for more, more, more than what they already have? What are men growing into? These Peter Pans shamelessly admit they don't want to venture out on their own.

Woke young people lack drive because everything is done for them. So, they embrace mediocrity and conformity. Reece Witherspoon's son attended college in New York. After he showed his posh pad to a friend, he was called the derisive term "Nepo Baby," or child of nepotism. While woke folks rally for "equity," they also interpret the word to mean "sameness"—as long as no one is more "same" than they.

Long before Prince Harry whined that his Royal heritage abused him, there were plenty of men around the world voicing legitimate unhappiness with how they were being mistreated as men. Men's complaints are usually whispered to protect them from being called "weak."

Gilda-Gram
Men struggle for a language of masculinity.

My First Experience with Men Who Didn't Stand Up

I saw male weakness first-hand when a Wall Street firm called on me to train its top managers to improve their interpersonal communications with their staff. I entered a dimly lit conference room and saw twelve men sitting at a long, imposing mahogany table. Their boss hired me to provide sound principles to improve the bottom line through the firm's human capital.

After greeting these men and assuring them that everything discussed in this room would be confidential, I asked, "How can I best serve you during the next two hours?" The group's responses took me off guard. Each man complained that his boss neglected to give him regular raises and promotions. I asked, "Have you shared this with your boss?" In one way or another, every one of them responded, "He should know."

I had to halt my prepared presentation. The next half hour was spent providing these men with a safe place to vent—and the venting was plentiful. Fortunately, they felt secure enough in my presence because they admitted this was the first time they could be truthful about their work grievances.

After the group spilled their frustrations onto the mahogany, I explained that their boss was not a mind reader, and each of them needed to communicate his needs. They agreed they felt uncomfortable expressing their weak-seeming feelings to their boss. I asked, "Why?" They said they felt that complaining could lead to a worse fate.

<u>**Gilda-Gram**</u>
**A situation won't change
until the lesson it's meant to teach is learned.**

Psychologist Abraham Maslow advised, "One can choose to go back toward safety or forward toward growth. Growth must be chosen again and again, and fear must be overcome again and again."

I laid out the only two options the men had: Become your own advocate, or continue to be "safe" but silently fume—and see no change in outcome. They were beginning to understand.

Next, I lowered the boom: "You're behaving like love-starved women awaiting Prince Charming to save you. Prince Charming doesn't know you even exist. Besides, he's desperately trying to salvage his hide from the sharks circling his monarchy."

I said, "Does your boss know your career goals? Does he know you're upset? He's been busy putting out fires because of the staff's low productivity. That's why he called me here today. Put yourself in his shoes."

After this unexpected empowerment session, I delivered the material I had prepared for our meeting, and the men were very receptive.

While traditional psychology focuses on the question, "What is your *problem*?" I believe it should instead ask, "Where is your *power*?" How quickly people grow with that question!

I left the men with this:

Gilda-Gram
Write your own comeback story!

The managers vowed to take the reins and tell their boss what they honestly wanted and why they believed they deserved it. In other words, they were now charged to sell themselves because they had a new belief in their talents and their brand.

Upon returning home, I began to consider that businessmen in our culture sit on a powder keg that could blow at any time. They fear seeming weak and inept, especially to the people who deliver their paychecks. Rather than share their feelings and look to iron out the kinks, they ignore their upset. Often, men self-medicate through sports, drinking, womanizing, and other excesses we'll discuss later in this book, but each is merely an escape and, at best, a temporary fix. Come Monday morning, discontent has festered because it was never probed and processed. It's no accident that there is an uptick in heart attacks on "Blue Monday" at 9 am.

Similar to the women I described to them, the guys thought their "prince" was their boss who would save them. Meanwhile, the boss had no idea his underlings signed him up for this role. I explained to the men that they were living a fairy tale. They didn't want to hear that.

After meeting with these guys, I felt compelled to write a book of anti-victim, take-charge skills called "Don't Bet on the Prince!" The book was meant for women because that's the gender that devours self-help principles, and if one gender becomes more assertive, so will the other. It was published in multiple languages in multiple countries, went into its second printing, and has since been called a "bible" by women who use it to guide them into healthy relationships. Because of its business-based principles, I also used it in New York as a business text for my graduate MBA students—women *and men*—to understand healthy communications.

Despite its seemingly feminine title, men in my classes continue to read it and have palpable epiphanies. One man brought the book to class covered in brown paper so people would not know what he was reading. But another male boasted, "This book is a chick magnet. I walk in the street with the cover visible to all, and women approach me for being such a sensitive guy!" Women appreciate sensitive men—as long as they sport a backbone as well.

Why is there interest now in understanding men's interpersonal communications? Our culture has lost sight of the things that matter—the soft skills—and how people can relate honestly and truthfully. We have identity problems that create trust issues. We've been preoccupied with designer labels and flashy cars to impress... who? And why? We've forgotten—or never learned—how to empower ourselves in pure and naked transparency. We've forgotten—or never learned—how to rise above the judgment of people who should not count. We've forgotten—or never learned—how to be kind. We've forgotten—or never learned—how to honor and respect each other. We've forgotten—or never learned—how to be sensitive to people's needs.

Recently, there has been significant focus on the LGBTQ+ arena, and this openness has made life for this group healthier than it's been. For 35 long years, Jodie Foster felt uncomfortable admitting to being a lesbian. In the shadows of her sexual preference, she welcomed two sons and had a thriving acting career. Barry Manilow admitted that hiding he was gay was a "burden," and he was always worried. In the 1980s, record producer Clive Davis explained that Elton John's career had been damaged after he revealed he was gay. Manilow kept his secret to himself, as did Foster, so their careers could prosper.

Whose business is it to know with whom we sleep? It is awful to try to live life and achieve success under oppression—and these are two who survived the scrutiny. Many others succumbed to the pressures.

Today, being gay seems commonplace. But now, as though *the culture always needs some group to hate*, discrimination has moved to heterosexual men.

Sherita Hill Golden, a black chief diversity officer at Johns Hopkins Medicine, named all white people, heterosexuals, Christians, and men as "privileged" because they derive "unearned personal, interpersonal, cultural, and institutional benefits at the expense of others." Golden's statement was met with a storm of fury, including from the richest white heterosexual man on earth, Elon Musk, who tweeted, "This must end!" A humiliated Golden apologized, "I retract and disavow the definition I shared, and I am sorry."

But the white comedian Chelsea Handler had chimed in two years earlier that "White men's opinions are pretty irrelevant." Joy Behar on The View summarized former President Trump's attempted assassin as another of the many "young, white men with guns." Her remark went viral, and she took heat for it. But in reality, school shootings ARE mostly white boys "acting out their hopelessness," in Warren Farrell's words.

Farrell continues, "Boys who hurt us are boys who hurt." Their self-esteem hurts from being told to pick between "woke" and "toxic," without an alternative safe place to go. Rather than treat their pain, society skips many steps and goes straight to punishment.

Farrell notes, "The commerce of masculinity is the trading of wit-covered putdowns." If a guy can't take the heat in a "joke," he's ridiculed. The bias against men—and white men in particular—can turn to trauma. Now we learn that 14-year-old Georgia school shooter Colt Gray was bullied by peers who called him "gay." In addition, his dad called him a "sissy," "p--sy," and "bitch" because he believed that his son was too gentle. These "wit-covered putdowns" were no joke to this kid. He snapped and shot the AR-15-style rifle his father gifted him for Christmas to man him up. He killed four people and injured countless others. After the massacre, Colt trumpeted, "I did it."

"Watch what you say," I advise my media coaching clients. I caution them to think carefully before "Open Mouth, Insert Foot" sets in. Once they're out, words—and the biases that spurred them—can never be erased. Sherita Golden will not be able to redeem her racist reputation. And thanks to her ill-conceived and unfiltered hatred, an esteemed medical school was stained. When will this hatred end, and along with it, the rampant idea that anyone can utter hurtful epithets without repercussions?

Hetero men are mocked by exclusionists like Golden and Handler as well as by their own families and the media. They remain mired in confusion, with rusted and flaccid rudders, as they try to navigate the waters of life and love, self-medicating their way through perilous behaviors that extend from withdrawal to uncontrolled rage. It is no wonder that women are asking where they can find a solid guy who likes who he is. With all the put-downs, a guy won't be proud of who he is. A man who likes who *he* is can like who a woman is and enjoy healthy, trusted, and lasting interaction!

Albert Einstein declared, "Intellectuals solve problems; geniuses prevent them. We need our men—and our women, too—to *prevent* dysfunction *together* before it takes us all down! While "Don't Bet on the Prince!" spoke to women, "Real Men Don't Go Woke" speaks to men.

PART I

MEN'S NEW FEELINGS

In a new age of relaxed traditional gender roles, both genders are confused and suffering. The Internet compounds the consequences. In the past, fury toward someone meant expressing your frustrations but not causing bodily harm. Today, vindictiveness has ballooned, and getting viciously even with an enemy, is becoming the norm.

Sun Tzu's "The Art of War" teaches not to toxically outshout but to intelligently outsmart, a perpetrator. Observers should hear rage as rage, but also and especially as pain.

A hurting population can't love and be loved. A hurting culture cannot be economically sustained. Hurting heterosexual males have been called malignant and toxic by people who don't see their confusion. Phil McGraw brilliantly noted, "It used to be that people would talk about 'toxic masculinity.' Now, they talk about masculinity as toxic. I think somebody needs to stand up and talk about that." Thank you, Dr. Phil. Yes, and that's why I wrote this book.

Warren Farrell points out that male toxicity emanates not from the perception of a man's power and control, but from *the suppression of his feelings of vulnerability*. So, while the culture has appropriated the term "toxic male," its true significance is a man's power*less*ness to express his emotions. When a man stuffs his power, the result is anger, which Farrell names "vulnerability's mask."

But here's today's problem. When we express our feelings, people turned off by our words cancel us. Cancel culture makes our divides even more cavernous. Bari Weiss of The Free Press gave a TED Talk in April 2024 called "Courage, The Most Important Virtue." She blames this culture of crisis on the cowardice of the closeted, self-silencing majority.

Of course, speaking up makes a person vulnerable. Many men think that vulnerability is a curse word. Country music singer Brandon Davis shatters that myth with his lyrics, "Tough don't mean you can't cry." Tears have healing properties, and to hold in sadness makes a person sick, fat, and/or depressed.

Dr. Phil stepped out on a ledge by criticizing the toxic masculinity movement. I stepped out on a ledge by writing and titling this book as I did, despite the top book publishers refusing to publish this topic. Weiss says, "Cowardice is more contagious than Covid. But so is courage" if we choose that path instead. Yes, it takes courage to disagree in public, but the cowardly woke won't even disagree. Instead, they chop opponents out of their arena.

A woke gay friend I had for decades spoke about his voting preferences during a phone conversation. I told him I wasn't voting the way he was. He immediately cut me off, although I had no qualms about continuing our friendship. A year later, he texted me, "What happened to us? Was it politics?" He didn't even recognize that *nothing* happened to us from my perch. The problem with wokesters is their unwillingness to consider dissenting views.

Good friend of Taylor Swift, 18-year-old Brittany Mahomes, wife of Kansas City Chiefs quarterback Patrick Mahomes, liked a post on Instagram that said "Trump-Vance 2024." The couple comes from a Texas town that leans Republican. Brittany is a Sports Illustrated model, former college soccer player, and mother. Fans of Taylor condemned the like. Brittany responded, "To be a hater as an adult, you have to have some deep rooted issues you refuse to heal from childhood." She continued, "You can disagree with someone, and still love them. You can have differing views, and still be kind."

Bill Maher noted that now the two friends won't sit in the same box at the Kansas City Chiefs game. He remembered how they sat together for every game last season. He asked, "Don't you think partisanship has gone too far?" Swift had denounced Trump. As with my woke gay friend, have politics between these females ruined their friendship?

Agreeing with Sun Tzu, Weiss concurs, "We don't solve our conflicts with blows. We solve them with words." Brain power is communicated through words. The head of TED,

Chris Anderson, pointed out the issue: "The tools of words are often heard as an assault."

So, if we are unwilling to hear each other's words, where are we going as a society? Weiss correctly warns, "The line between civilization and barbarism is paper thin." Love and compassion are only possible if we agree to be civilized. "People who claim that words are violence are taking away the most fundamental tool we have for virtues like courage," Weiss concludes.

Males who feel disoriented and misunderstood should not need to take cover. Instead, they should be empowered to express their truth. George Orwell said, "During times of universal deceit, telling the truth becomes a revolutionary act." And that requires courage to speak up.

Nation Cymru, a news magazine from Wales, says, "There are Black History Months, Women's Disability, various race and religious history months, and soon, LGBT+ History Month. Every year we hear, 'Why isn't there a white men's/able-bodied/straight and so on, history month?'" Author Norena Shopland responds that history is dominated by able-bodied white heterosexual men independent of diversity, so there's no need to celebrate them. *What?*

Today, men are even punished for being ordinary and healthy. A British woman, Karie Jane, moved to Spain to open a nude resort. She says "pervs" who don't cover their erections are escorted off the premises and banned from ever returning. She says that those who accidentally engorge will not be disciplined as long as they cover up and are subtle about their bulging member. Everyone is required to sit on a towel and close their legs. *Some vacation!*

One Quick Fix for the Male/Female Disconnect

John Burn-Murdoch outlined new research in the Financial Times as a potential reason men and women are finding difficulty connecting deeply: they're split on a widening political chasm.

In the U.S. and Germany, women between 18 and 30 are 30 percent more liberal than their male contemporaries. In the U.K., the gap is 25 percent. Moreover, King's College London found that young men are becoming more conservative! In the midst of cancel culture, if a guy isn't in a woman's lane, she cancels him! Yet, I continue to get "how-do-I-find-the-one?" questions from young women unable to land love. *Let's open our eyes!*

Burn-Murdoch said, "In the wake of the #MeToo movement, young women have become more progressive and vocal about their views. Young men, however, feel threatened and have reacted by taking the opposite position." Why must we make politics the central focus of identity and a barrier to potential co-mingling? Goldie Hawn is a Democrat and her partner Kurt Russell of 40+ years is a Republican. Their romance has thrived despite their different politics.

When I hear a single man classify a new female prospect as

"not my type," I ask where his type has gotten him so far in his life. To save themselves from debilitating stress, I tell unhappy males to write a letter to themselves describing the issue they are suffering. When they see their issue in print, they can react to it as a problem to be fixed. When a woman is complaining, the man jumps in to rescue her with his fix. Women like that men are expert fixers. When a man re-reads his own letter days later to determine if the same issue still gnaws at him, he can adroitly devise change techniques. Or he can accept the situation as it is and end the self-flagellation. The fix requires observing, confronting, responding, and welcoming new positive energy.

Anger for men is the encouraged go-to behavior. When under duress, men don't usually employ their problem-solving ability. Instead, they express themselves as Wounded, Banished, Shamed, Unneeded, and/or Angry. Each of these behaviors drains their health and relationships.

Sun Tzu

"There are five dangerous faults:
Recklessness, which leads to destruction.
Cowardice, which leads to capture.
Delicacy of honor, which leads to shame.
A Hot Temper, which is provoked by insults.
Oversolicitude, which leads to worry and trouble."

All five of these "dangerous faults" are seen in current times, but men camouflage them to self-protect and hide from the pain that may accompany taking a stand.

CHAPTER 1

Wounded

When Will Smith was a vulnerable 12-year-old, he wanted to rap. He creatively wrote rap lyrics, and he shared them with his grandmother. Instead of reinforcing his proud endeavor, she was shocked that the words were expletive-rich.

Grandma wrote her grandson a follow-up critique: "Dear Willard, truly intelligent people do not have to use words like these to express themselves. Please show the world you're as smart as we think you are. Love, Gigi." After that missive, Will vowed to never again rap with curse words.

The problem with Will's vow was that curse-less raps are plain vanilla to the rap community, lush with obscenities. Soon after, Will won the title of being "soft." When David Letterman asked him if he felt pressure to quit music, Smith responded, "Not pressure as much as it was always that I was soft. I hated that, being called soft."

That statement reflected the deep scarring the young rapper

had endured from his peers. If he was willing to reveal this to Letterman and the world, didn't he reveal it to his wife? The demeaning "soft" title still ran through his veins, although he was grown and married with kids. He closeted his feelings of inadequacy while he shined in movies depicting other characters.

<u>Gilda-Gram</u>
A man may avoid conflict to keep peace,
but he starts a war inside himself.

Certain words can be emotional triggers for men. The word "soft" is one of them. Is it any wonder my training those male executives on Wall Street in "soft" skills met with resistance?

An unknown male on a social media video ranted, "And for the few real men out there in Western society, stay hard." Yes, men universally intuit that they must never be considered "soft." This warning carries through to male sexuality. Observe the plethora of male enhancement products available to maintain that symbolism of unbreakable masculine toughness, being HARD!

A YouTube ad for Baerskin pitches a "tactical hoodie." The announcer growls, "The average hoodie made these days is weak, flimsy . . . You're not a child. You're a man." Such is the message from the other side of wokeness.

Everyone on the planet was dropped on his head, and nobody completes childhood without wounds. Why aren't we giving our men leeway to be human—and demonstrate softness AND hardness? Why must it be one or the other? No man should feel discarded, devalued, disrespected, or wounded for who he is.

CHAPTER 2

Banished

To avoid conflict, many males hang out on the corner of Peace-at-any-Price. They rationalize that they would rather pick their battles, or they choose to wait out a storm. But onlookers who observe men being trounced on or bullied deem them as gutless. These men wonder why they've been banished from further interaction. They often let it go—until at the wrong place, the wrong time, and with the wrong person, their bottled-up emotions burst. Eventually, feelings must have a place to go!

Kanye

The world watched as Kanye West argued with ex-wife Kim Kardashian on Twitter about being banished from their children's lives. Kanye has bipolar disorder, and when he takes his meds, he functions better than when he does not. But he doesn't like how he feels when he takes them, so he often doesn't bother. No matter what his mental state was at the time, however, the one steady issue Kanye continued to argue for was the care of his four children with Kim.

In caps, he tweeted, "SINCE THIS IS MY FIRST DIVORCE, I NEED TO KNOW WHAT I SHOULD DO ABOUT MY DAUGHTER BEING PUT ON TIKTOK AGAINST MY WILL."

Kim tweeted back, "Kanye's obsession with trying to control and manipulate our situation so negatively and publicly is only causing pain for all."

Further, "Kanye's constant attacks on me in interviews and on social media is more hurtful than any TikTok North might create."

Declaring herself North's main provider, Kim continued, "I am doing my best to protect our daughter while also allowing her to express her creativity in the medium she wishes with adult supervision."

Kanye recoiled, "What do you mean by 'main provider'? America saw you try to kidnap my daughter on her birthday by not providing the address to the party. You put security on me inside the house to play with my son, then accused me of stealing. I had to take a drug test after Chicago's party 'cause you accused me of being on drugs."

He continued, "Let me get this straight. I beg to go to my daughter's party, and I'm accused of being on drugs. Then I play with my son, take my Akira Graphic Novels, and I'm accused of stealing. Now, I'm accused of putting a hit on her. These ideas can get someone locked up."

The post's title by the unknown author who detailed this interchange read, "This is what post-separation abuse looks like. Using children as pawns to manipulate, control, and threaten a parent." I didn't perceive Kanye's interaction that way. Was he "manipulating, controlling, and threatening," or just wanting to participate as a parent in his children's lives? Men caught in the crosshairs of divorce and child-rearing understand Kanye's chaos too well. They want to be fathers with a say in their child's upbringing, not banished as mere sperm donors.

Brad Pitt was caught in the same estranged-parents/children-choosing-sides dilemma. A headline in the New York Post concluded that "Angelina has already won the family war." Pitt was "devastated" when one-child after another legally dropped his last name. He hopes that when they're older, they'll think for themselves.

Suri, the daughter of Katie Holmes and Tom Cruise, dropped her father's last name. Is this cancel culture trend the way children egged on by their moms get back at their dads? While the dads feel banished, their dad-deprived children may suffer abandonment issues, which could manifest as anxiety, distrust, and relationship problems. These kids could eventually seek love in dangerous ways.

When men feel banished from their children's upbringing, they lose a significant part of their being. Moreover, so do their children for lacking their paternal role model. Banished men are angry for being treated as familial window-dressing.

Will

This world-renowned actor kept his feelings of banishment in his relationship under wraps—until he exploded during what was supposed to be a celebratory ceremony.

On March 27, 2022, at the 94th Academy Awards, Chris Rock was on stage presenting for the Best Documentary Feature. As he entertained the audience, the laughter was contagious. In one joke, Rock addressed Will Smith and his wife, Jada Pinkett Smith, who was sitting in the audience. He said, "Jada, I love you. I can't wait to see you playing GI Jane. (Jada shaved her head because she suffers from the autoimmune disease, alopecia areata, where sufferers lose their hair.) Jada rolled her eyes at the joke, but husband Will, sitting at a right angle to her, laughed exuberantly.

Out of sight of the cameras, Will registered Jada's disdain. Smith reformatted his laughter into anger in a split second and steamed onto the stage. He shockingly slapped Rock in the face with an open hand. The celebrity-filled audience thought it was part of Rock's act. But when Smith returned to his seat, his profane shouting warned Rock never to mention his wife again. The audience froze.

All eyes were on Rock's next move. Calmly, the comedian remained on stage. A few seconds later, he said, "Oh, Wow! Will Smith just smacked the sh-t out of me." And soon, he joked, "That was the greatest night in the history of television." The audience unfroze and laughed as Rock continued his presentation without missing a beat.

At first, viewers worldwide thought this was part of the act. But they slowly began to recognize they had witnessed an assault. Yet, true to all things Hollywood, construction grips were already setting up the next scene as soon as the curtain went down on that set. Without one mention of what had transpired earlier, the 94th Academy Awards presented Smith with the Best Actor trophy. The audience vehemently applauded, and the slap was momentarily forgotten. Smith apologized to the Academy of Motion Picture Arts and Sciences and the other nominees in his acceptance speech. There was no apology to Rock.

The next day, Smith did apologize to the comedian on social media and again to the Academy. The incident went viral and generated so much buzz Smith was forced to resign from his membership in the Academy, and he was banned from attending Academy events for ten years.

Williams' 23-year-old son, Jaden, didn't see a problem with his father's actions. The millennial smugly defended, "This is how we roll."

Gilda-Gram
Children model themselves after their parents.
50 percent of our learning is set by age 5.
30 percent more is set by age 6.

A year after The Slap, Jada Pinkett Smith began promoting a new book. She told the world that during the Oscars, she was shocked that Will called her his "wife." The pair paraded themselves as husband and wife, but now the public discovered that for the last seven years, the Smith Family merely played the roles of a happy tribe to be emulated by all. Jada explained they'd been separated all that time. The joke was on us.

This family's pretense affected not only onlookers. The Smith "celebrispawn," Willow and Jaden, had also been directed to perpetuate the lie of being perfect. The kids didn't cause their parents' issues, they couldn't cure them, and they couldn't control them. Being helpless, their burden was great. Their inability to be kids left them traumatized during their sensitive teen years. In their twenties, they began to act out.

Jada was desperately trying to sell her book no matter how many carcasses she mutilated. She was putting her wants before her husband's needs, but this was probably nothing new. Will had become Jada'd many years before. Was he too woke weak to leave?

Throughout history, men have given away their power to women to get female approval, probably starting with Mom. But grown women crave a man who stands his ground.

Jada took public humiliation to new monetized heights. Ana Navarro on The View said this was Jada's money grab: "Every time she needs to sell books, she drops these bombshells." Her co-host, Alyssa Farah Griffin, slammed Jada for "oversharing" intimate details of her marriage and not being in tune with her husband's feelings. Saturday Night Live ridiculed Jada with a caricature that said, "If we got divorced, he could mess around and end up happy. And I can't have that."

In real life, oblivious Will rationalized, "We have had a very, very long and tumultuous relationship. We call it 'brutiful.' It was brutal and beautiful at the same time." SNL corrected that term to be "brunhealthy," a mix of brutal and unhealthy.

Jada discussed the couple's "deep love for each other." Her critics chimed that someone with "deep love" would not humiliate her mate every chance she gets. Didn't she realize that Will's character reflects on her own for choosing him? While searching for headlines to make the news, she didn't care who got hurt by her revelations, including her kids. She unabashedly revealed she never wanted to marry Will, and she only did because she was pregnant with Jaden, thereby also humiliating her son, who heard he was an unwanted accident, now fraught with keeping his parents together. Recognizing that his household was less than savory, Jaden tried to become an emancipated minor at 15 when his parents secretly separated. Reflecting the rest of her questionable parenting, Jada introduced her son to psychedelics. It was later feared that he was self-harming with dangerous drugs.

Daughter Willow was mortified by her mom's airing of the family's dirty laundry. She said, "Growing up in the spotlight is excruciatingly terrible." Jeers from her peers left her with depression. She cried for help on social media, "You either quit or keep going. They both hurt." Did her mother see this desperate post, or was she buried under her pretentious book promotion?

Meanwhile, Jada whined that Will's Slap cost HER the loss

of her Red Table Talk Show on Facebook TV She complained that people were calling her an "adulteress" and that she was the one getting punished. She wanted Will to find a new home for her show. But because of The Slap, Will no longer had clout in the industry. Is that why she and her daughter Willow, who was on that show, became angry with him? Or were they angry at him for being weak? Smith became a lifetime member of "The Doghouse." Some women enjoy taking advantage of weakness, but most women become bored with all that manipulation.

Despite all his flaws that Jada was quick to enumerate, she said she's not divorcing Will. Her net worth is $50 million, while his is $350 million. The lifestyle façade is too attractive to leave, although, with his uncertain future, he's trying to save money despite her excessive spending.

Loral Langemeier, author of "The Millionaire Maker," accurately writes, "Most wealth is inconspicuous. The man down the street driving the nice car and living in the mansion could easily have greater debt and a lower net worth than the wealthy plumber who drives a beat-up truck but seems to work only when he doesn't feel like fishing."

Gilda-Gram
Happy people aren't consumed by material consumption.

If their conspicuous wealth is depleted, will Jada still have that "deep love" for her husband? There is a healthier way to live besides bigger-better-more.

To add insult to the already deep injuries she had carved, on her show, Jada shockingly discussed with Will her affair with her son's friend, twenty-one years her junior. She demeaningly called it an "entanglement" before changing it to "relationship." Fans were angry that she blindsided and humiliated Will. My National Enquirer column on Jada as a man-eater received about 100,000 responses on social media from fuming fans.

Instagram comments about Will's narcissistic wife were, "She's definitely got something on him since he won't leave her and her abusive emasculating;" "Please delete this couple from the Internet;" "Does he have Stockholm Syndrome?" –the condition where hostages develop a psychological bond with their captors.

Jada humiliated her husband and took down the "other man," August Alsina. His response to his involvement in the Williams family drama was to release an angry collaboration titled "Entanglement" with rapper Rick Ross: "You left your man just to f--k with me and break his heart." Alsina has been seriously ill with a debilitating autoimmune disease, but to Jada, he's another fallen cadaver to be abandoned and banished.

Further humiliating Will, Jada named deceased rapper Tupac Shakur as her "soulmate." And to boast about her desirability, she bragged that Will hit on her while he was still married (thereby making *him* the adulterer, not *her*!), and Chris Rock asked her out on a date. Could these put-downs get uglier? Rock told Jada to keep his name out of her mouth.

Yet, Jada arrogantly predicts that she and Will probably will live together one day again. Will is 55, and Jada is just two years younger, but she told The Today Show's Hoda Kotb, "Will is getting old." "Old" is a damning word in Hollywood, so that was another put-down. "Who's going to be there for him?" she asked. "It's going to be me."

The 2021 HBO-MAX documentary "15 Minutes of Shame" asks, "What does disproportionate shaming do to a person? To the shamers? To society? There is a human price to be paid, and its currency is PTSD, depression, and anxiety. Andy Warhol's famous 1968 quote was, "In the future, everyone will be famous for 15 minutes." In medieval and renaissance times, shaming consisted of being sentenced to the pillory. Historical shaming has been replaced by exposure on social media. And it seems to be encouraged by "Schadenfreude, The Joy of Another's Misfortune," the book title by Tiffany Watt Smith. It's sad when "damage joy" becomes empathy's replacement!

So, Jada humiliated Will, Jaden, and August, the men closest to her. But trying to destroy her husband, only to be his savior when he's old and impaired, could assign her the diagnosis of Munchausen by Proxy. She would get the credit for his salvation while she was the one who created the condition.

Jada needs psychological help before she destroys any more male lives. In a somnambulistic state, Will insists that Jada is his best friend, and he will show up for her and support her for the rest of his life. Or is it until the end of the rolling credits or the credit cards?

Dear Will Smith,

The person who makes a difference in our life is not the one with the most beauty or the most awards. It is the one who cares about us the most and shows it, not in words, but in behavior. Ask not, "Do I love *her*?" Instead, ask, "Do I love *me*?"

Dr. Gilda

Yet, despite what everyone tells anyone to do,

<u>Gilda-Gram</u>
Every person is and will remain
where he wants to be.

Healthy people will not stay in a relationship that feels like a maximum security lockup. The choices are to change the relationship or change the behavior. A union is only good as long as it works for *both* people. If it breaks down for one, it will break down for both.

The Slap proved that Will isn't doing well. Author Carolyn Myss says we know our contract with someone is complete when that person can't hit our hot buttons any longer.

A poster of a great-looking guy on social media says, "I don't walk away to teach people a lesson. I walk away because

I learned mine. I'd rather adjust my life to your absence than adjust my boundaries to accommodate your disrespect."

* * *

One Isolated Slap Can Cause an Avalanche

After The Slap, renowned comediennes voiced fears of lawlessness on their stages. Less than two months later, a copycat rushed Dave Chappelle on the stage of L.A.'s Hollywood Bowl. The attacker pulled out a replica gun that could eject a knife blade. When the assailant started running, a mob chased him, caught him, and put him in the hospital, where he was arrested.

Chris Rock, who performed a set earlier in the evening, joined Chappelle onstage and joked, "Was that Will Smith?"

During the curtain call, Jamie Foxx stood beside Chappelle.

Foxx told the crowd, "Listen, this man is an absolute genius. We've got to make sure we protect him at all times." And to Chappelle, he said, "We're not going to let nothing happen to you."

Tyler Perry felt torn because of his friendship with Smith and Rock. He said, "It was wrong in no uncertain terms." After the incident, Perry described Smith's reaction as "stunned, not really understanding what had happened." Perry sorrowfully declared, "To get all the way to this moment, winning an Oscar, that was one of the crowning moments of his career that he wanted so desperately. I think he is trying to figure out what happened."

Gilda-Gram
**People who feel unworthy
validate their unworthiness in their behavior.**

Will Smith remained out of the spotlight for the following year.

CHAPTER 3

Shamed

Shame expert Brene Brown says, "If you don't claim shame, it will claim you." She names the hurt that is behind pissed-off, shut-down men. She says that men think women would rather see them die in battle on their white horses than watch them fall off as losers. For men, shame is a failure in their profession or status or money, being wrong, being defective, being soft, being sexually dysfunctional, and showing fear. (Women feel shame through body dysmorphia.)

There are three ways of coping with shame:

1. Disconnect from others.
2. Move against others in anger.
3. Move toward others as a people-pleasing doormat.

The Problem with People Pleasing

Sun Tzu
"Peace proposals unaccompanied by
a sworn covenant indicate a plot."

People pleasers are needy for love. Children try to please their parents and link their self-esteem to external rewards. Adult people pleasers struggle to provide self-care without guilt.

The disease to please employs winning favor by kissing ass. But they are caught off guard when they find the ass they kissed was the wrong one. Leland Val Van De Wall said, "The degree to which a person can grow is directly proportional to the amount of self-truth he can accept without running away."

Gilda-Gram
**People don't need to like you
and you don't need to care.**

An exponent of the "Don't-Blame-Me" mindset, people pleasers tend to blame others instead of themselves. Symptoms of shame are the same as those of trauma. The pre-frontal cortex goes into fight or flight mode.

Psychiatrist Daniel Amen says chronic brownnosers can metamorphose from dejected to respected by adopting self-discipline. He tells people pleasers to only do nice things for people who treat them respectfully.

Paula dated a people pleaser a few times. Each time after they saw each other, he would vanish. Then she received this text: "I know you think I have disappeared. And I guess I have. I'm letting you know I am okay. I have been very introspective, and I'm sorry if my disappearance has hurt your feelings. It's not my intention. I'm still not ready for any relationship with anybody at this time. I enjoy your company very much, but I feel guilty because I think you like me too much, and I just feel empty inside. I don't wanna hurt your feelings or anybody else's anymore by continuing to pull away from people. So, for now, I'm just gonna go to work and come home. Read a lot of books at night. I'm sorry."

Paula responded, "Thank you for letting me know you feel empty inside. I don't know why, so there's a lot you've hidden from me. I can't have a relationship by myself. I know we connected deeply, and I wonder why you made overtures if they had no basis in truth. Without transparency, there is no relationship. I can't be with a man who is not honest. This appears to be your pattern, and I don't do chorus lines. Get help or continue your pain."

He wrote back, "I'm very sorry."

How could this guy be sorry if he could not "feel"? An insecure and narcissistic guy would not seek help because he is terrified of uncovering his true feelings. His state of misery allows him to capitalize on his comfortable "poor, unlucky me" victim stance. This people pleaser admitted to Paula he was slowly letting down his guard. Maybe that, too, was a lie.

"Women Can't Hear What Men Don't Say," is the title of one of Farrell's books. Apology accepted, access denied.

* * *

The perfect example of camouflaging shame as rage, or as Brene Brown might put it, "pissed off"-ness, was the Will Smith Slap. According to a 2022 Gallup book, "Blind Spot: The Global Rise of Unhappiness and How Leaders Missed It," people today feel more anger, sadness, pain, worry, and stress than ever. Every breakdown in every sector of business and personal life reflects this unhappiness.

Of the 7.7 billion world citizens, since 2006, only one in five claimed to be enjoying a great life. What does the 20 percent of the population have that the miserable 80 percent do not? Gallup's definition of "happy people" credit being fulfilled by their work, having little financial stress, enjoying their community, maintaining good physical health, and sustaining loving relationships.

Misery cannot be hidden for long. To rectify the mood, without professional credentials, numerous celebrity "rescuers" sporadically offer advice to the masses. In June 2022, Chelsea Handler said it was time for her to be a voice for women on late-night television. Guest-hosting for vacationing Jimmy Kimmel, she said, "Nobody can experience being a woman other than one of us. White men's opinions are pretty irrelevant."

This view is shared in corporate America. A white hetero male was applying for a corporate grant for his small business.

On the form, he was required to check his ethnicity. The categories read "African American," "Native American," "Hispanic," and many he had never heard of. There was no category for "Caucasian."

Handler fancied rebooting her E! talk show, which ran from 2007 to 2014. However, there seemed to be no bites in television land. She later complained to Variety about the disinterest: "It's the same white man problem. There are too many white men doing the same job." Despite Handler's assertion, Gallup does not mention the proliferation of "white men" among their five concomitants of happiness.

Fox News analyst Gianno Caldwell, whose younger brother was murdered in Chicago in June 2022, complains that liberals demonize him, a black male conservative. Liberal Handler only mentions *white* males. Whatever their color, full-bodied heterosexual males are not in high regard in current times. Why don't men of all colors revolt against being demonized?

Joe Collins, a California congressional candidate and U.S. Navy veteran, answered what has happened to today's males. Seeming like a replay of 1835 with Washington Irving, his video says that weak men are the downfall of America.

> "America has a problem with men. Not regular men, but with the punk ass, soft ass, feminine ass, beta ass, gossiping ass, crybaby ass men. You guys never argue with logic. It's always some feelings-type crap. It's

always 'I feel like this' and 'you're hurting my feelings.' These are extreme feminine ways. Pick your nuts up and start acting like men. You guys are men. I don't care about what they tell you about toxic masculinity. You guys are toxic feminine. If you disagree, write, 'I disagree' and state why. Nobody gives a damn about your feelings."

Women complain about not being able to find men with backbones! Women say they want sensitive men—but guys better not be overly sensitive. How do we measure "somewhat sensitive, but not overly so"?

A Gen Z 27-year-old woman went out with a 35-year-old man. Afterward, he texted, "Hey, had fun last night. Have a good day." She wondered if he wanted to see her again. Instead of asking *him*, she posted his private message on social media for 500,000 people to decipher! Fearful of a woman's rejection, men default to communicating in non-committal fashion and women also afraid of rejection won't ask for clarification. Instead, they run to groupthink to try to figure it out! Neither gender communicates honestly with the other.

Hailey Paige Magee, author of "Stop People Pleasing—and Find Your Power," says, "One way to hone our boundary-setting and honest communication skills is to practice inserting a *space* between a trigger and our response to it." Thus, replace knee-jerk, people-pleasing *reactions* with intentional, assertive *responses.*" Instead of looking for group approval, the 27-year-old woman should have directly told the man she wanted to see him again, and asked if he felt the same way. If Will Smith had taken Magee's prescribed pause, history would have been different.

* * *

Another Complication for Men: The Honey/Money Ratio

From the beginning of time, men sought honey, and women sought money. One guy advertised on an online dating site, "I would like a loving, considerate companion to shower with affection and clothing." *Clothing?* The honey/money equation perpetually puts the Mr. on the make and the Ms. on the take.

The Mouths of Innocence
Question: When is it okay to kiss someone?
"When they're rich." –Mary, 7

Thomas Pollet, a psychologist in Australia, found that the pleasure women derive from making love is directly linked to the size of their partners' bank account. The wealthier the man, the more frequently his partner has orgasms. Ahh, so size counts after all—but it's the size of a man's wallet. Ladies chant, "Girls Just Wanna Have Funds." But to preserve mental health, money-hungry women should differentiate between a guy's net worth and their own self-worth.

Embodying the Honey/Money Ratio, Crystal Hefner, Hugh's third wife for five years, admitted she had never loved the guy and had been "brainwashed." She was 30, and he was 86 when they wed. To promote her new tell-all book, she said it wasn't easy sleeping with an 80-year-old. Instagram fans pounced on her for using the word "brainwashed" to appear as a victim.

"American Idol" winner Ruben Studdard met Surata Zuri McCants in 2006 when signing CDs in Atlanta at a Walmart. He followed her around the store until they made contact, and in 2008, they were married. After two months together, however, she discovered he had major money problems and no record deal in sight. By 2012, the marriage was kaput.

It's hard on guys who lack loot. In New York's tony Hamptons, penniless playboys were combing through trash cans at bank ATMs looking for receipts with big account balances. When they met an impressionable girl at a club, they put their phone numbers on the backs of the bank slips. The girls who fell for the ploy deserved the paupers they ultimately got.

Prince Andrew's ex-wife Sarah Ferguson dated Norwegian businessman Geir Frantzen, who gave her a Bentley! There may be a reason the wealthy guys I knew never even gave me a toy car. The University of Michigan found that the more intelligent the woman, the less impressed she was by a man's wallet. Wise women earn their own money and don't need sugar daddies.

The Honey/Money ratio is a silent language between men and women. As we walked past a high-end dress shop, a man I casually knew said, "You'd look great in that dress. Let me buy it for you." I refused, knowing there would be an expected but unexpressed exchange for my gratitude.

Newly minted divorcees have not yet become fluent in the Honey/Money language. A recently divorced Tracy Morgan lamented, "I keep meeting [bleep]ing gold diggers . . . a chick wants to spend all my money up—and then gives me a hassle when I want her to [bleep]."

* * *

Needy men are too myopic to see destructive women. A lawyer in a top New York law firm was earning millions, and he and his wife and kids were living "the life." But he had a heart-attack kind of job, and he finally told his wife he was quitting. She quickly divorced him. He painfully concluded, "She only wanted me for my money." To not know the woman to whom you've been married for 12 years describes the superficiality of the relationship. The lawyer had been so enmeshed in making money he did not fathom the lack of love under his roof.

The pains from marital dysfunction are deep and dangerous. Its remedy starts with examining and knowing who you are to assess a partner accurately.

How Will I Impress?

Gilda-Gram
**A man can't say the wrong thing
to the right woman.**

Insecure men worry about how they come across, and they shame themselves for not being "enough"—rich enough, successful enough, smart enough, buff enough, hard enough. What will it take until they feel good enough? Alison Faulkner writes, "Enough is a decision, not an amount." When a man decides he is enough as he is, his quality interactions expand.

In California, 37-year-old Rob Mercer tried to raise $10,000 to enter the World Series of Poker Main Event, the world's most prestigious poker happening. He told people he had terminal colon cancer and set up a GoFundMe page. The phony victim raised between $30,000 and $50,000 and was allowed to enter the tournament. When questioned about his illness, Mercer offered vague responses and failed to provide concrete proof of his diagnosis. Finally, Mercer came clean. He said he *believes* he does have "undiagnosed" breast cancer. He said he created the colon cancer story because breast cancer is usually a woman's disease, and he didn't want the humiliation of aligning with a female disorder. The fear of seeming weak motivated this man to concoct a more *manly* disease!

On a special episode of "Real Men," Pastor Mark Driscoll, Trinity Church, Scottsdale, Arizona, said, "In the eyes of God, one of the worst things a person can be, but particularly a man, is a coward."

Sun Tzu
" . . . recklessness leads to destruction,
and cowardice leads to capture."

Little boys are told, "Big boys don't cry," "Man up," "Don't be such a baby," or "You throw a ball like a girl." As grown men, they try to conceal their imperfections. I wear an obvious white sensor on my upper arm to monitor my diabetes numbers. A man in a store asked about it as his wife stood silently beside him. He confessed that he should be wearing one himself, but he's "too afraid" to see his blood sugar levels. How ironic that men boast to be fixers, yet when problems concern their health, they won't fix themselves!

Mary's husband suddenly died while they were on a trip to Ireland. Her grieving involved rage because he had not taken care of himself while he still could. Craig had diabetes for years, but he avoided exercise at all costs, sneaked candy bars at his desk, and sprawled on his couch at night watching movies. He had suffered a few strokes, got a few heart stents, and had two toes amputated for gangrene. Now that he was gone, Mary retraced how Craig had been cavalier about his health. The two of them had gained 50 pounds each because of their inactivity. She told friends, "I won't be his nagging mother." Now, she was angry she had not mothered him after all.

Melanie had lost her husband three years earlier to prostate cancer. Upon his death, Melanie learned that he had not once gone for a PSA test, the assessment for prostate cancer. She moaned, "How could he not have taken care of himself?"

Both women fumed over their husbands' self-neglect. But like the diabetic husband in the store who admitted he's "too afraid" to learn the truth about his blood sugar numbers, both husbands chose to bury their realities. Neither of their wives was willing to treat their husbands like their sons. Neither man is alive today.

It is well-reported how men avoid medical care unless their women nudge them. Andrew Gould, former Arizona State Supreme Court Justice, wisely said that a large percent of life is failure. But "it's not failing that makes you a man. It's how you respond to it."

CHAPTER 4

Unneeded

A significant source of depression in men is caused by no longer feeling needed, which William Farrell calls the "purpose void." Feeling unneeded makes a man feel worthless. Deeming himself an "extra" in his family constellation, the younger son of King Charles III and Diana, Princess of Wales, Harry is fifth in the line of succession to the British throne. Grieving his mom's untimely death at 12 years old and suffering PTSD and anxiety afterward, the once happy-go-lucky Harry titled his memoir, "Spare," to denote an unneeded part. Many men today perceive they are unnecessary. Farrell notes, "the psychology of masculinity is the psychology of male disposability."

In the 2009 movie, "Not Easily Broken," characters Dave Johnson and his wife, Clarice, appear to have it all. But consumed by her career, Clarice puts her husband's needs on the back burner. Dave laments,

"In the old days, women saw their men as conquerors, providers, heroes. But somewhere along the line, it changed. Women started becoming their own heroes. Maybe it was because their men forgot how to be heroic. Or because women didn't want to be protected anymore. Or maybe women had to be their own heroes because of the pain they endured. But whatever the cause, the world took away a man's reasons for being a man. They told him he wasn't important anymore."

Years ago, I asked male college students how they would feel if their wives made great money. They applauded the prospect without exception—but with the caveat, "as long as she doesn't make *more than* I do!" So, it would be okay for a female partner to be empowered as long as her power didn't overshadow her mate's.

Collette Dowling's 1982 book, "The Cinderella Complex: Women's Hidden Fear of Independence," and later, my book, "Don't Bet on the Prince!" applauded empowered women. However, some women on dating sites still conceal their success to avoid intimidating male suitors. Medical doctor Marilyn calls herself a nurse. Trial attorney Allison describes herself as a paralegal. If they meet a man they like, the ploy continues for the same reason. Does a Real Man want an untruthful woman who deflates her value to inflate his? Eventually, that inflation goes flat.

Feeling the heat of competition, Travis Kelce bought a $6

million mansion to impress his new love, Taylor Swift, after feeling "self-conscious" that his life lacked his lady's kind of opulence. Compared to Swift's residences, a mansion Travis's size is a drop in the bucket. Brothers Jason and Travis Kelce signed a new podcast deal with Amazon for $100 million, which will bolster Travis's net worth. Still, will the love birds' imbalanced finances cause friction over time?

In 2012, designer Vera Wang had been married to Arthur Becker for 23 years. The pair were known for berating each other publicly, making onlookers uncomfortable. For many couples, fighting is a form of foreplay. Becker had been a former CEO of a tech firm, not exactly a lightweight. Yet, he resented being regarded as "Mr. Vera Wang," assigning him an inconsequential role.

The ex-husband of Jimmy Choo founder Tamara Mellon told W magazine, "When your wife makes $100 million during your marriage, it's quite a shocker . . . I felt like my masculinity had been stripped from me. I felt like my b--ls were in a jar."

What would my former male college students say about a Madge-Pays-Guy reversal of tradition? Guy Ritchie got $70 million in his divorce from Madonna. When they married, he already had a name and wealth. The couple knew they were economically mismatched from the start, but as with the exes of Vera Wang and Tamara Mellon, it's tough on a man when his woman's wallet is more gigantic than life.

But then there's the Queen of Real Estate, Barbara Corcoran, whose net worth is $100 million. She is married to Bill Higgins, a former Navy Captain. The disparity in their earnings seems to have no bearing on their 40-year marriage *because he is secure in knowing who he is.*

When 44-year-old Theresa told her husband of five years, Fred, that she wanted a divorce, he acknowledged, "You don't need me anymore. You don't want my name, you don't want my babies, and you want to earn your own living. You just don't need me."

Theresa tried to explain that she never *needed* him for those things. She told him she *wanted* him as an equal emotional partner in their marriage and life. This was a concept that he—and most of his friends—could not fathom. The traditional male template has been to be needed as a father to their kids and a financial supporter of their family. But not as an equal partner. Fred later confessed he had a "hero complex."

Motivational speaker M. Curtis McCoy wrote, "Men want to be the hero. We want to solve problems and treat you like a princess. Constantly complaining makes your guy feel like he's the reason you're not happy. When this continues, we distance ourselves from you and the relationship."

When single, Fred would get involved with women of low economic and academic status to "save" them from the lifestyle they were "enduring." Each relationship elevated him to warrior in charge of the pair's future. Not understanding his previous romantic debacles, he was now experiencing another relationship disintegration with Theresa.

A man with a hero complex ties his self-worth to the

behaviors of a woman needing to be saved. Some women don't want to be saved, so no heroism is needed there. Others complain that the "saving" does not come with enough perks, so no heroism is needed there, either. Still others may initially sign up for a quick "my-hero" swoon (*ahhhh*) but soon feel incarcerated by *too much* saving because it chokes them. That was Theresa.

Without a person to save, what is a hero to do? The "You don't need me anymore" phrase that Fred used was correct—but not because of the *things* he said his wife no longer needed from him. As two equal spouses, Theresa wanted *emotional* support, friendship, companionship, and partnership. Although Fred remained in the dark, it didn't matter because he quickly moved on to save a damsel in real distress.

CHAPTER 5

Angry

When anger is turned inward, it becomes depression. At other times, the anger is out there for all to see. Anger is always based on fear. Native American Chief Red Eagle said, "Angry people want you to see how powerful they are. Loving people want you to see how powerful YOU are."

In Houston, Texas, two men viciously beat up and robbed a confused Spanish-speaking 67-year-old man with Alzheimer's and dementia when he mistakenly tried to get into their car. The frail man pulled on the locked door handle. An unwatchable video showed how the thugs stomped on his head viciously and repeatedly punched him. The rage these criminals displayed over this minor mistake suggested it had been percolating inside them without an outlet until they found this ready victim!

Men will share their anger but never the hurt beneath it. Our culture has made it too humiliating for males to admit the scrapes of humanity. In contrast, women feel energized when they spill their feelings to their besties. For all their football kind of huddling, men will stick together and cover for each other, but women, after their teary togetherness, might turn on each other. Which behavior is less healthy?

A joke on the Internet exemplifies men's and women's different views of friendship.

> **Friendship among Women**: A woman doesn't come home at night. She tells her husband she slept at a girlfriend's house. The husband calls his wife's 20 best friends. None of them know anything about it.
>
> **Friendship among Men**: A man doesn't come home at night. He tells his wife he slept at a friend's house. The wife calls her husband's 20 best friends. Eight of them confirm he had slept over, and two claim he is still there!

As depicted in the joke, the aftermath of The Slap reflected a tight male cabal that honored the brotherhood. While it is understandable that an impressionable son would defend dad Will's crime, was Jamie Foxx advocating to "protect" Chappelle by having that cabal put more attackers in the hospital? Sun Tzu posits that physical violence should only be the last resort.

Some males on my LinkedIn page argued that it was appropriate for Smith to defend his woman's honor the way he did, while others condemned converting anger into assault. Thus, men had differing views of how to combat perceived verbal attack.

Sean Penn weighed in, "I don't know Will Smith. I met him once. He seemed very nice when I met him. He was so f--king good in 'King Richard.' So why the f--k did you just spit on yourself and everybody else with this stupid f--king thing?"

After The Slap at the 2022 Oscars, Smith was still allowed to accept his first Oscar. Penn angrily fumed, "Why did I go to f--king jail for what you just did? And you're still sitting there? Why are you guys standing and applauding his worst moment as a person?"

<u>Gilda-Gram</u>
The issue we see
is never the real issue.

Smith's famous assault prompted rare discussions among men. The talk was about Will and Jada's open marriage, the state of men today, relationships, confrontation, verbal assault, violence, the defense of a lady, and anger.

It was open knowledge that Will and Jada were non-monogamous. Will was ribbed in Hollywood about his loose marital status. It had to be especially humiliating that Jada discussed with Will her infidelity on her show. Will became a ridiculed cuckold living in the unforgiving celebrity fishbowl.

<u>Gilda-Gram</u>
Whatever you don't change,
you *choose to continue.*
Whatever you choose to continue
is rewarding you in some way.

The Bible's Samson & Delilah reveals how a woman betrays a man. A strong warrior with superpowers, Samson was blinded by love for his wife, Delilah, who he chose among the Philistines with whom he was at war. She married him just to discover the secret of his strength, which she evilly planned to reveal to her people. Deeply besotted, Samson succumbed to Delilah's urgings to divulge that his hair was his power source. While he slept, his wife cut off Samson's mane to suppress his strength.

Traditionally, long hair was a symbol of masculinity. The Greeks wrote odes to heroes' hair: The longer the hair, the more manly the warrior. And following the story of Samson, when a warrior was captured, his mane was cut to humiliate him and diminish his power.

As soon as Samson lost his strength, the Philistines attacked him. But by the time they readied him for prosecution in the town square, his hair was beginning to grow back. With that growth, his force returned. A superpower again, Samson was able to demolish the temple, killing himself and the Philistines. But this freed the Israelites from Philistine rule, so Samson lost his life and became a historical hero.

Not unlike Samson, Will Smith had been traumatized by his wife's public brutality. Since Will had suppressed his feelings for years—the seams of his tolerance suddenly burst at the most damaging time of his career.

It is easy for actors to bury their emotions. Entertainers legitimately depart reality each time they perform as characters. I posit that all actors have some form of DID, Dissociative

Identity Disorder, so they can separate who they are in real life from the characters they play. As a great actor, The Slap proved that Will lives his art while he avoids his life. He never figured out where to go with his pain.

Some men take their pain out on women. A new dating craze, "stealthing," finds angry men using a condom when the mood hits, only to remove it without telling their partner. When women find they have been exposed to potential disease or pregnancy, some are psychologically traumatized.

In 2019, researchers found that men who removed condoms without consent were more likely to have had a sexually transmitted infection or have had a woman suffer an unwanted pregnancy. In 2021, California became the first state in the United States to make it illegal as a civil offense, although not criminal. Vermont, Texas, and Utah are considering passing anti-stealthing legislation based on California's precedent, but progress is slow because of disagreement over whether stealthing should be regarded as rape. As of May 2023, laws or precedents against stealthing exist in Germany, Australia, Canada, the Netherlands, Switzerland, the United Kingdom, and New Zealand. Stealthing reflects the height of men's anger against women.

Another angry expression of men towards women is "pump-and-dumping," or fleeing the scene the moment sex is done. This makes a woman feel like the guy's "personal masturbatory sleeve," said sex expert Nadia Bokody. The sexpert emphasizes that no woman wants to feel like a "discardable object."

A healthy solution to anger is acknowledging hurt as soon as the first arrow pierces the heart. But that would require a departure from the reactive Cro-Magnon lunge.

Most people are not adept at coping with thorny issues, at least without professional guidance. Males who stuff their feelings inside rather than seek therapy miss out on developing the coping skills needed to navigate hostile environments throughout life.

I often ponder whether the universe intentionally wounds us to push us to grow. "Acting" in a healthier way does not include or excuse "acting *out*." The 1987 movie, "Broadcast News," encapsulates when someone is about to take a stand: "I'm mad as hell, and I don't want to take it anymore." Despite its noisy reaction, the movie exemplifies how anger can drive a new and healthier resolution.

The ability to understand, interpret, and control emotions is called "EQ" or "Emotional Quotient." While we can't control what's happening, we can control how we respond. Daniel Goleman's 1995 book, "Emotional Intelligence" popularized the concept. Some experts argue that EI is inborn, while others say it can be learned and strengthened.

With so much violence in our culture, it is evident that the level of EQ has declined. Peaceful communicators have higher EQs than those who rage with fisticuffs. Yet, the media highlights and thereby encourages the blood and gore through its reporting.

* * *

I was the Relationship Expert on the 2013 Valentine's Day Special, "50 Ways to Leave Your Lover" on Investigation Discovery TV. The show depicted bizarre lover-leaving triangles. Viewers frighteningly watched real people invite the word "anger" to be prefixed by a Capital "D" in "**D**anger." Budda says, "You will not be punished FOR your anger; you will be punished BY your anger." If a relationship is not nurtured, intimacy will collapse. People desperately try to prove they're loveable by creating new adventures with another person. If those adventures are secret, that adds to the intrigue—but beware.

Here are two stories of love triangles that turned dangerous. The first was televised on Investigation Discovery, where I, as the relationship expert, explained the behaviors.

He Left His Wife to Have a Child with Her Friend

In Dallas, North Carolina, Tabatha Johnson and Wade Logeais had a lot in common when they met: hot sex, foamy beer, speedy NASCAR, and truck stop trysts. Tabatha was a stripper, which titillated Wade's fantasies, and the pair became inseparable, traveling the country on Wade's truck deliveries. Soon, they decided to marry and begin having the many children Wade wanted.

Studies show that strippers accentuate their physical

attributes while their interpersonal relationships suffer. After giving birth a few times, Tabatha longed to prove she still had what it takes. She returned to stripping, but now, Wade objected to this profession for his wife. He suddenly demanded a more respectable partner. Tabatha rebelled against giving up her "profession" just because Wade told her to. Like a defiant adolescent, she chose to stay out every night, drink, drug, and leave her husband alone with the kids, causing ferocious fights.

Tabatha tried to repair the damage by bringing strippers home to Wade. Statistically, 85 percent of males fantasize a ménage a trois, but only six percent get their wish. Friends coined Wade, "a lucky guy," but he now decided he longed for a traditional marriage.

Like other misguided marrieds, this pair reasoned that having another kid would improve their relationship. Tabatha negated having one more pregnancy. Since she and Wade were accustomed to threesomes, they asked Patty, a woman from their trailer park, to become the baby mama. After giving birth, Patty agreed to hand off the new baby to Tabatha like a dirty diaper.

The plan backfired when Wade fell in love with Patty, who mothered his child. For revenge, Tabatha put an icepick in her husband's face, she left the scene, and Wade and Patty married. However, within a few years, Patty ran off and left Wade alone with the large family he said he always wanted.

* * *

Husbandly protectiveness is not unusual. When Kanye West was married to Kim Kardashian, he told her he didn't want her to dress sexy, despite that her brand before they met dripped with sex, exploding her fame through her highly publicized sex tape. West and Kardashian fought over the way Kim dressed. When he tried to control her, she rebelled. After they divorced, he chose a new wife, 28-year-old Italian Bianca Censori, who was compliant. His different standard of propriety consisted of "dressing" her in mostly invisible clothes.

West divorced a starlet to dazzle with a harlot! He deliberately paraded Bianca and her banging body around the world almost nude! Kanye (or Ye) forbade her to speak and wear certain clothes, eat special food, and work out, even though he didn't follow the same standards. The pair traveled like conjoined twins. Together, they attracted worldwide attention, which was the ego-builder Kanye apparently needed.

Women often lose themselves in their partner because relationships are women's dominant love language. In some, a trauma bond can evolve. "Stockholm Syndrome" describes the psychological affection of a hostage with her captor despite the harm inflicted. Issues of dominance, submission, superiority, and inferiority trigger mental illness.

Despite her seedy lifestyle, Tabatha from the Investigation Discovery show refused to become a manipulated Bianca Censori.

He Ignited Their Love Nest

In New York City, forty-five-year-old Wei Chu Wu was furious at his wife, Yan He Zheng, the mother of his 13-year-old son, who he believed was cheating. A neighbor whose child played with Wu's child in the park remarked that this seemed like an average family. But the two argued angrily and loudly.

In a rage, Wu's irrationally set fire to their entire apartment building. The five-alarm flames engulfed all the floors, killed one of the building's residents, and injured seven firefighters. But the real object of Wu's wrath, his wife, escaped with their son. Was the anger worth it?

When anger rules, nobody wins.

PART II
NEW WORLD CONDITIONING

With increasing numbers of women frustrated that men are too weak, many woke men profess they're feminists and feign respect for women. On the surface, that trait seems attractive. But one woman complained, "I will never trust a self-proclaimed male feminist again. The man who has to tell you he is king is no king at all; they don't respect women." Other women chimed in with stories of being raped and assaulted by their so-called feminist guy friends.

One woman wrote, "Working in a heavily male-dominated field, I learned to trust the men who called me 'Toots' and outright told me 'Women don't belong here' over those who acted woke and buddy-buddy. The former were honest; I knew where they stood and could bluntly call them out. The latter were quickly offended by the mere *idea* that they weren't God's gift to women, and they were quick to stab me in the back." Another added, "Often the people who positioned themselves as 'on my side' were the most bigoted and sexist once they started opening up with their true opinions—to the point of openly belittling me and invalidating my experiences when I disagreed with them."

Woke men do not always win popularity contests. Shannon Ashley titles an article, "What Can We Do with All These Broken Woke Men?—A Plea to Start Talking." She calls out the faux feminine come-ons dipped in syrupy placation so they can get closer—for texting or sexting. Many young women are apparently onto this cloak of woke that conceals a man's true intentions.

Why can't a guy just boldly state his intent? The answer lies in the properties of wokeness: gender roles are confusing, and "macho" has become an expletive. So, a guy may deliberately err by spouting feminist doctrine.

If wokeness continues to cancel all the stuff it doesn't like, where is the diversity of thought that these groups advocate? A staffer for Maryland Democrat Senator Ben Cardin, 24-year-old Aidan Maese-Czeropski, recorded 8 seconds of himself having male-to-male intercourse in his workplace, in the same room Supreme Court nominees are grilled. Sure, he was fired, but instead of apologizing, he claimed the Right was targeting him because he's gay and a Democrat.

Being woke also means playing victim. But continuous "Woe is me" mantras get old after a while. In 2019, Democratic President Obama warned against wokeness: "You should get over that quickly." How many people listened?

CHAPTER 6

Masculinity's Numerical Score

In 1980, Geert Hofstede, Ph.D., a Dutch social psychologist, identified six dimensions of cultural values in more than 50 countries. One of the dimensions was masculinity. He explained that "masculine cultures" value heroism, competition, and achievement, with men proud to boast of their status and success. In contrast, feminine cultures value cooperation, modesty, and caring for those in need.

A country's high masculinity score suggests gender differentiation, where men assume the traditional roles of strength, courage, leadership, and assertiveness. This value system begins in childhood and continues throughout life. Masculine cultures typically work long hours and take little vacation time, as earnings and achievements take priority over family life.

China is considered the world's most masculine country,

scoring 66. The masculinity score of the United States has been considered high, with a score of 62. However, Hofstede's data are now being criticized as outdated. Increased female independence, LBGTQ+ influences, trans lifestyles, the declining emotional health of men, and the blurring of differentiated gender roles between males and females have led to "feminized" males that are leaving men themselves confused.

In the United States, developmental psychologist Gary Barker found that almost 50 percent of young men say they think about suicide frequently. Two-thirds of young men said, "No one really knows me," which Barker calls a cry about loneliness. To cope, men close themselves off to human connection by saying, "I don't care." You can't shame, question, hurt, or embarrass them because *they don't care*. Barker says we need to talk to boys and men about how they *do* care, nurture, and love. Once closed off, suicide, binge drinking, bullying, traffic accidents, depression, and sexual harassment of women continue to rise.

Chemical Exposure

Researchers continue to probe why men have lost their masculine edge. Studies have shown that the Y chromosome, which determines the male sex, is gradually shrinking. This Y chromosome has lost 900+ of its genes over the last 166 million years, and in about 11 million years, it might completely disappear. Might these findings relate to sexual dysphoria, or the distress a person feels when his gender identity doesn't match his birth sex?

RFK, Jr. blames chemical exposure for sexual dysphoria, especially in boys. He reports that the chemical atrazine is put in our water. He says that if we insert that into a tank of frogs, it will chemically castrate and feminize them. "Ten percent of the male frogs will turn into fully viable females able to produce viable eggs," Kennedy cautions. "If it's doing that to frogs, there's other evidence that it is doing it to human beings," he warns.

Isolation

Another reason for the loss of masculinity may be modeled after the Japanese custom called "Hikikomori," which describes people, many of them men, who are in isolation. Low testosterone is one of the signatures of these young social recluses.

Just A Poet Guy posted on the Internet: "One of the hardest lessons I've ever learned is that I stayed in so many dark places because I believed I deserved to be there when I didn't." Quite an admission, but at least he had the epiphany.

Political economist and author of "Men without Work," Nicholas Eberstadt, suggests the United States practices a version of Hikikomori with seven million men of prime working age jobless and apathetic about wanting to change that status. They choose to be indoors playing video games, watching porn, and indulging in drugs. This behavior is especially concerning since the testosterone levels of young American men have been plummeting for years, affecting one in four.

Is making men more feminized intentional? Director James Cameron announced that testosterone is a toxin that must be flushed out. There have been discussions about the association between "toxic masculinity" and testosterone. However, science has not linked high testosterone with aggression and violence. Yet, low testosterone in men is associated with social anxiety and submissiveness. The Cleveland Clinic further associates it with depression, brain fog, and an inability to focus clearly. Research at Emory University demonstrates the influence of testosterone on the hypothalamus, which is responsible for creating oxytocin, the bonding hormone that prompts couples' togetherness.

A study done in 2017 found that male gamers had lower libidos than other men. The researchers suggested that engaging with video games released dopamine—the same "pleasure hormone" released during orgasm—which could contribute to disinterest in sex with a real person.

Sun Tzu
"Concentrate your energy and hoard your strength."

Young bucks act like they'll always have what they have now. It will be a shock when they find out otherwise, which could lead to even greater depression.

Porn

Another culprit of lost masculinity is porn. A study of men aged 18 to 68 found that higher porn usage sees poor body images and eating disorders as men try to model the bodies they see on screen.

And now we learn that new research from MarketWatch Guides finds that Gen Z aged 19 and below are more interested in tech than tires. They are opting not to want to drive, thereby disavowing the traditional teenage rite of passage. A lot of these young men would rather stay in and connect to their porn and video gaming.

Israeli professors Ateret Gewirtz-Meydan and Zohar Spivak-Lavi found that the greater a man's relationship with porn, the more likely he is dissatisfied with his body and more vulnerable to eating disorders. Their research studied heterosexual, homosexual, and bisexual men. The United States is seeing a rise in both eating disorders and body dysmorphia in young men, along with an increase in young men who watch porn. Psychiatrist Dr. Carlos Chiclana in Spain expanded the connection between porn and negative body image to both male and female heterosexuals.

Active porn use also increases erectile dysfunction, which accelerates shame. A 2020 study published in the Journal of Urology found that there is a correlation between the amount of time spent watching porn and the amount of time it takes to reach orgasm.

Testosterone levels are also plummeting among young men who watch porn. The Cleveland Clinic found low testosterone in about two percent of men. Symptoms include depression, impaired sleep cycle, loss of body hair, reduced libido, erectile dysfunction, and low sperm count. A 2017 study found that gaming also releases dopamine, the same pleasure hormone released during orgasm. If gamers are getting off with their games, they're less interested in intimacy with a live partner. Moreover, the stress gamers experience combined with the excitement similar to sex depletes testosterone.

A 22-year-old male admitted, "I wasn't motivated to actually pursue a real relationship or even talk to women because I was getting my fix through porn." He was unable to sexually function in real life after watching the acted excitement of the professional performances on screen. These dysfunctions mainly affect millennial males who grew up with unbridled access to the Internet.

Meanwhile, competing with the airbrushed porn images, Gen Z females are seeking labiaplasty, or "designer vaginas," to win back the young men whose attentions are consumed by their screens.

According to a media poll, the average young man encounters porn first at age 12, and 58 percent find it unintentionally. One young man said that going cold turkey with his porn addiction reinstated a happy and real sex life and increased his social interactions.

Pornography can even be hazardous for the actors in this

profession. Australian porn star, Dani Dabello, brought her pet python to work on her porn set. Her sex partner wanted to meet eight-foot-long Betty, so Dabello draped the snake around his neck. Suddenly, the snake was biting the actor's penis, and blood was spurting as he tried to free his projection from the snake's mouth. Dabello checked to ensure Betty didn't leave her little teeth on the man's love machine as pythons often do after biting someone. Dabello claimed Betty had never bitten anyone before. But Betty was not the only snake attracted to men's appendages.

A 47-year-old man on a South African safari needed reconstructive surgery on his penis after a cobra bit it and it began to rot. A Tai teen on the toilet reading his smartphone was hospitalized after a snake bit his member. *Who knew that snakes have penis envy?*

Any man wondering whether his porn perusal is an addiction needs to answer three questions:

1. Am I spending time and money on kinky content preventing me from achieving life goals?
2. Am I watching porn in risky situations?
3. Am I substituting porn for real life relationships with real life women?

Any or all of these may be warning signs that require professional attention.

A form of cinema therapy can be found in the 2013

romance/sci-fi movie, "Her." A sensitive writer is heartbroken after his marriage blows up. He drops out of living by having an imaginary love affair with his computer's operating system. Her voice reveals a playful personality that continues to occupy him—until she crashes and burns. Men who view this film will watch the devastating damage that can occur when a man loses himself to fantasy.

Sex Dolls

Many men striking out with women eventually chuck the idea of finding someone to love. If they can't find a Bianca Censori, Kanye's obedient wife, they design a lifelike submissive doll according to their own specs!

Depending on what someone wants to spend, eerily realistic sex dolls can smile, moan, blink, get goosebumps, and even hold a conversation. Made of silicone, they look and feel like real humans. Some are part robot and can simulate a woman's orgasm. Bill Maher joshes, "Never make love to someone you have to unplug to clean."

A manufacturer's website describes, "There are lonely middle-aged men who don't necessarily want to stroll through the dating minefield again, there are handicapped and disabled folks for whom sex dolls are convenient and non-judgmental companions, and there are couples who wanna add another dimension to their love life without emotional baggage." One of these sexy dames can set a person back upwards of $6,000.

The Bedbible Research Center collects data on issues of sexology and relationships. It conducted what they term "the most comprehensive statistical study on sex dolls that has ever been done." It aggregated the purchasing data from eight of the biggest sex doll retailers with production data from three of the biggest manufacturers. The findings showed that 9.7 percent of American men over 18 own a sex doll. That's almost ten percent of men over 18 who prefer a fantasy to a real-life female. Are these the same guys who watch porn? The study noted that $3 billion worth of sex dolls are sold annually in the $37 billion sex toy industry.

During COVID, the sex doll appetite shot up 75 percent as a partner alternative, making 2020 a record year for the industry. What are those men doing now that COVID is over? Are they still isolating with their doll as much as young boys are glued to their video games?

Australian author Caitlin Roper wrote "Sex Dolls, Robots, and Woman Hating." She calls lifelike replica women and girls produced for men's sexual gratification "the literal objectification of women." Men commission the creation of their ideal woman from actual photos of *children*, and they can specify body type, breast size, skin tone, hair color, and more. They are sold on Amazon and Etsy.

Roper warns, "The dolls appeal to fantasies of pedophilia in child abuse scenarios. A popular video showed a man having sex with a child doll modeled on an infant." In Australia, childlike sex dolls are deemed a form of child abuse material that can result in ten years in prison and/or a fine of up to $555,000.

But now, women are getting equal opportunities. Bill Maher tells us someone is working on a male companion to the female robot with a huge bionic penis that ejaculates face moisturizer from Sephora. If guys felt inadequate earlier, wait till "Henry" hits the market!

Identity Unknown

An additional factor in lost masculinity is men whose identities are not grounded. At the 2022 Oscars, Will Smith's affect changed from laughter to fury in a moment when he barreled onto the stage to slap Rock. A Prayer for the Stressed says, "It takes 42 muscles to frown and only four to extend your middle finger and tell someone to bite me!" Men who are steadfast in their identity and have a high Emotional Quotient can respond without a tantrum and fists. Men whose identity is shaky become reactionary from cues from an outside source.

Hofstede updated his research in 2001, but we need new masculinity scoring with our more recent cultural add-ons. By 2010, the term "toxic masculinity" was being used to include physical and sexual aggression, violence, emotional control, power, and bias toward people who aren't heterosexual. The term "hegemonic" masculinity further legitimized men's dominant position over women and weaker men. So, the original Hofstede template for heroic, competitive, and triumphant masculinity had become tarnished.

Someone on the Internet commented, "Masculinity isn't toxic. The absence of it is. Weak men are abusive and angry. Strong, masculine men are protective and loving."

Chinese American conservative political commentator and former Miss Michigan Kathy Zhu commented, "Single mothers raise forty-three percent of boys, and seventy-eight percent of teachers are female. So, close to 50 percent of boys have 100 percent feminine influence at home and 80 percent feminine influence at school. Toxic masculinity isn't the problem. The lack of masculinity is." In 2019, just one day after Zhu received the Miss Michigan crown, she was de-throned. She bristled that it was more challenging to come out as conservative than it would be to come out as gay.

Like Zhu, actor Kevin Sorbo says that once he became vocal about his conservative politics and faith, he became "the original cancel-culture guy." He wrote a Christian children's book, "The Test of Lionhood," for youngsters to learn to celebrate masculinity. The book tells a story about a lion family, where little sister Chloe gets cut by a poisonous plant. Big brother Lucas must save the day.

Lucas can only save Chloe's life by getting a flower at the top of a mountain. He must overcome his fears, worries, and obstacles to climb that terrain. But through his ordeal, Lucas learns the meaning of real lionhood that incorporates bravery and perseverance.

Sorbo said he aims to wake the lions in America from being sheep and wake up Hollywood. He said he's on a mission like Mark Wahlberg and Taylor Kitsch, who are sick of the woke world.

Reflecting the strength of his demigod Hercules series in which he starred for six seasons from 1995 to 1999, Sorbo commands boys to be brave and manly. He said, "They shouldn't be afraid to confront dangerous things."

Sadly, another male actor chose suicide over that lion's kind of fight that Sorbo describes. South Korea's Lee Sun-kyun, the star of the Oscar-winning movie 'Parasite' was found dead in his car. "Parasite" was the first non-English-language movie to win best picture in the Academy Awards' 92-years. It was also the first South Korean movie to win an Oscar. In 2021, Sun-kyun won a Screen Actors Guild award. This guy was going places!

Now, he faced an illegal drug probe that South Korea strictly enforces. A drug violation in that country can result in six months in jail or up to 14 years for repeat offenders and dealers. Lee Sun-kyun shamefully said, "I am sorry for my family, who are enduring extreme pain at this moment." He was only 48. He left behind a wife and two children. Too bad he didn't choose to fight--either the drug charges or an addiction if he had one. Suicide is a coward's way out of shame.

A documentary on YouTube called "Why Movies Need Masculinity" complains about the movies' depiction of men. It called out men who try to one-up each other. The documentary reminisces that men in movies used to be fathers, friends, fighters, lovers, and leaders with respectful principles they always observed. It noted, "When confronted with loss, they would face their feelings and pick themselves up and move the f—k on . . . acting like a grownup. That's a man." Men learned from their mistakes and grew as people.

How did the manly movie character disappear? According to the documentary, violence in the 60s changed everything. Begun by Eastwood and Bronson and advancing to Stallone and Schwarzenegger, the manly man was a man of action. The overall message was that a lifetime of violence leads to emotional trauma. Tony Soprano ended up in therapy.

During that time, I had an Italian plumber who wouldn't take payment from me in exchange for my giving him private therapy to model what he saw on the Sopranos. This macho man would never have consulted a therapist before he watched Dr. Melfi work with Tony! Then it was okay.

The documentary points out that everything related to toxic masculinity, like aggression, heartlessness, selfishness, and abuse, is the stuff of the immature, not of the man. It laments that movies don't teach men to be men anymore.

CHAPTER 7

Softness is for Sissies

A would-be politician was running for a high office that required tough leadership. Despite advanced degrees and years of related work, he was short, pale, slight, and had a high-pitched, squeaky voice. One woman mocked that his handshake felt like "a wimpy grip from a skinny boy." This man brought incomparable credentials and experience to this competitive political race. But his non-verbal presence and projection screamed "soft."

Of course, not every candidate for office can be a tall, robust heartthrob. At one of his rallies, a male supporter effused, "I always thought John was 'soft,' but after working with him, I discovered he is tough as nails!"

There was that word again: "soft." Despite glowing qualifications greater than those of his opponents, John lost the election, and his constituents lost out. Soft men don't rate!

Somehow, the bias against vulnerable men has reached kids even in elementary school. Nine-year-old William Gierke wanted to raise awareness for breast cancer. He wore a pink t-shirt to school with the words, "Tough Guys Wear Pink." He felt proud to support the cause. But when the kids at school saw his pink shirt, they called him "sissy." William went home crying and didn't want to return to school. But a wise male teacher ended the bullying by donning a pink t-shirt himself the next day.

Even merely *suggesting* that a man is "less than" can be a blow to his ego. While in New York City, the usually mild-mannered Tom Hanks felt compelled to transform into a protector of his wife, actress Rita Wilson, when a crowd of fans practically knocked her down. Hanks screamed, "My wife? Back the f–k off! Knocking over my wife?!" Tom's anger seemed to be out of character from the impeccably respectful reputation he has in Hollywood. Yet, four months earlier, his 30-something drug-addled son, Chet, publicly proclaimed he did not have a "strong male role model" growing up. That must have crushed his dad. Was Tom Hanks now over-reacting to defend his wife because of the earlier threat to his reputed male role modeling? No one knows how deeply male pain can go.

Stanford Professor Benoit Monin says that when a man's masculinity is threatened or trashed, he will try to recover by using exaggerated aggression and hostility. These "recovery" methods are often poorly thought out and become reactionary. Luis Umanzor, a 49-year-old New York man, faked being kidnapped to try to re-entice his estranged ex. Had he analyzed this ploy, he might have realized that he probably would have scored more street cred with his lady if he had *been* the kidnapp*er*!!

Twenty-five-year-old Tyrese Haspil was a personal assistant of a tech CEO. Greedily, he stole $400,000 from his employer to impress his French girlfriend. His boss had kindly seen Tyrese as his protégé, so when he discovered the missing money, he declined to press charges and arranged for Tyrese to pay him back in installments. However, Tyrese continued to steal from his boss. He was again discovered. Fearing being prosecuted, now he worried that his girlfriend would leave him. Believing his boss would testify against him, he reasoned he only had two choices: suicide or homicide. He chose the latter. He forced his way into his 33-year-old boss's $2.4 million apartment, tasered him, and then stabbed him to death.

His girlfriend must have left anyway, because when the police picked him up, Tyrese was on the street with a new girlfriend who he was showering with gifts. He tried to impress his women with grandiosity that was not his. Since the cultural group to eviscerate now is heterosexual men, the most insecure among them will try the hardest to impress.

The father/son background is crucial to a man's development. One man lied about being a Vietnam War vet when he had never fought in that war. He wanted his dad to be proud of him. But after his father died, the son was shocked to learn that his father, too, had lied about his military service. This son had wasted most of his life trying to live up to his father's glory. But the glory never existed. The fear of being weak, soft, and insignificant motivates the need to embroider macho narratives. When will men be proud of who they are *as they are*?

CHAPTER 8

But Macho Has a Price

R. W. Connell describes "hegemonic masculinity" theory as the general standard for a "Real Man." In our culture, it legitimizes men to exercise dominance.

Hegemonic masculinity values concealing a man's hurt emotions yet sanctioning him to act out his hurts. On hundreds of national TV talk shows on which I appeared, men cheating with other men's wives would be attacked by the husbands while their adulterous wives remained blameless! Each cuckold felt he needed to defend his masculinity so as not appear like a weakling.

Jose Gutierrez-Rosales, a 49-year-old Californian, was bullied at work for being a cuckold. He angrily defended his masculinity by killing the co-worker consorting with his wife. In another incident, Sean Armstead, 36, a New York City police officer, gunned down his wife's suspected lover and then killed himself. Is this the brand of masculinity we want?

Jack the Ripper was an unidentified serial killer in a poor

neighborhood in London, England, in 1888. He killed at least five poor women on whom society looked down. Is that the brand of masculinity we want?

Without provocation, on the streets of New York, men are punching random women in the face. One nose was bloodied, another was broken, and there were other unprovoked injuries. What level of anger would motivate this? Is that the brand of masculinity we want?

Rudolph Giuliani was the "tough-on-crime" mayor of New York. Dubbed "America's mayor," he irradicated the filth and corruption and pulled the city together after the attack on the World Trade Center. However, the world also rubbernecked into Giuliani's cheating on one wife after another and the very public familial nastiness that was exchanged. In his later years, with prostate cancer, public divorces, and estranged-children stories, he might have opted for a quieter life. But this lawyer remained ego-driven to stay politically relevant. He now has various lawsuits lodged against him. Is this the brand of masculinity we want?

In 1980, Alexander Haig became President Ronald Reagan's Secretary of State. When Reagan was shot, Haig demonstrated bold, masculine grandeur. True to the pompous pattern of his speeches for which he was often derided, he announced,

"Constitutionally, gentlemen, you have the president, the vice president, and the secretary of state in that order, and should the president decide he wants to transfer the helm to the vice president, he will do so. He has not done that. As of now, I am in control here in the White House, pending the vice president's return, and in close touch with him."

Haig received criticism for sounding like he was ready to lead the country, even though he was not next in line for succession. Twenty years later, in an interview with "60 Minutes II," he was still compelled to defend what he had said years earlier. The issue ruined the statesman's reputation. Even all those years ago, it was clear that when a man takes a misstep and is criticized, there is little room for redemption and evolution. The culture has forfeited compassion and forgiveness for heterosexual men. Is this the brand of masculinity we want?

Funnyman Will Ferrell makes us laugh while he pokes fun at himself. Married to the same woman since 2000 and father of three sons, his life appears mellow, although he's also part of the Hollywood machine. The tabloids don't write about Ferrell, except in his occasional declarations for the Democrats. Is this the brand of masculinity we want? Or would women find this kind of affable guy boring?

* * *

As they grow up, male and female roles are somehow programmed in young children. My nieces choose to play with dolls; my nephews choose to play with vehicles. When they're in a store, how do toddlers know what toys to select? I accompanied a friend and her 4-year-old son on a merry-go-round ride. At first, this little guy said he was anxious to mount one of the bobbing plastic horses. But once onboard, he rebelled with, "This is for girls!" The little tyke sulked by getting off the horse and standing *beside* it, not *on* it, while the merry-go-round continued circling. His mom couldn't imagine how he determined the horses were for girls! And why would that have made his participation demeaning?

In one of my MBA classes, I tried to explain how parents unconsciously raise their boys and girls with different gender standards. An outspoken father of two toddlers, a boy and a girl one year apart, vehemently disagreed, claiming he and his wife are absolutely and deliberately raising their two kids equally. I smiled and asked him to observe what was happening in his home.

When the class resumed the following week, my student described how his daughter and son played with other children in the sandbox as he and his wife watched. He noted that his wife said nothing when his son threw sand at another little boy. But when his daughter did the same, she was disciplined to "play nice." When her husband shared with his wife how differently each child was being disciplined, the mom herself was shocked.

I explained how the male stereotype of "boys will be boys" has been allowed to flourish, even and especially to the height of aggression. The dad apologized to the class and me and joked that his wife should be getting the three credits for our course because of all the parenting she's learning through her husband!

When boys grow into men, anger and hostility are more acceptable than they are for grown women. It's almost as though men's mantra has become, "If you get bitter, you'll be better."

Angry women are unattractive, while the culture applauds angry men as "tough." With this mindset, cowboy grit is the new swoon-worthy rage, reflected in the popularity of neo-western TV series like Yellowstone, starring Kevin Costner, and its offshoots. Yellowstone hit up to 11 million same-day viewers per episode!

Western-style cowboys are the tenacious testosterone-rich carnivores that many women are suddenly craving. A March 2021 Australian survey of 1000 men and women found that both genders associate meat-eating with "manliness." The survey found that 73 percent of men would rather live ten fewer years than go without eating meat. And 79 percent of these men vowed not to stop eating meat even if it would help their health and the planet.

There seems to be a correlation between the popularity of Yellowstone and the growing interest in professional bull riding. Sean Gleason, CEO of Professional Bull Riders (PBR), announced in January 2023, "Across three events this weekend—New York City, Portland, and Lexington—PBR had the biggest regular season weekend of ticket sales and attendance in our history!! He named this a "thundering start to our 30th anniversary season."

A reactionary return to Marlboro-man-masculinity is opposing woke weakness. Yet, hegemonic masculinity presents stressors on men's mental health. In 2019, The American Psychological Association issued guidelines for practitioners who work with men and boys. Psychiatrist and trauma expert David Reiss calls out "toxic competition" as the drive to win at all costs, regardless of who gets hurt.

An Internet joke asks, "Will 'Manwich' be forced to change its name to 'Gender Neutral Meat Sauce'"? The icon of macho requires gore to defeat the opposition, similar to a steak's bloody drippings. But at what price to men? The Marlboro Company's first owner died of lung cancer. So did the first Marlboro Man.

After the manhood of both Will Smith and Tom Hanks was publicly shamed, each was apparently driven by the need to reclaim his street cred. The drive for men to recoup feelings of adequacy is so strong that it might manifest in unrecognizable behaviors. I have observed men trance out in rage as they defend their point of view and identity. Sadly, their acting out often takes them to a place they cannot recall after their manic episode.

Scared by their capacity to lose it, many men don't realize they allow punctures to their identity to amass silently. I observed this behavior in that dimly lit conference room on Wall Street with the twelve angry male executives. When the upset can no longer be contained, like a warm bottle of champagne that is shaken, the cork pops—often at a place and with a person unrelated to the source of the hurt.

Within one week, I watched three successful grown men in diverse situations have vulgar tantrums over issues they had allowed to fester. These guys sustained the façade of confidence, success, strength, and composure to the world. But inside, they raged—until they exploded.

According to Mental Health America, depression affects six million men. Since the pandemic, men's depression increased by 154 percent. Perhaps it's because men define themselves by their work, and "work" as they previously knew it was defined as some mystical place away from home. Now working remotely, men become more visible to their families, detracting from their mystique.

Depression is a disease that doesn't get enough press. In upstate New York, 51-year-old Christopher Wood told his estranged wife, "This is how it ends for us," and then shot dead his innocent 14-year-old daughter before shooting himself. His estranged wife described him as depressed. In Austin, Texas, 43-year-old and three-time Emmy Award-winning actor Billy Miller died after battling depression. He had a brilliant career on the soaps, "All My Children," "The Young and the Restless" and "General Hospital."

Finally, some well-known males have courageously shared their stories of shame about their depression. Ignoring inevitable judgment, these men are finally willing to declare, "I'm imperfect."

Former "American Idol" judge, 63-year-old Simon Cowell, admits to having been embarrassed to seek therapy for his depression. He rationalized the traditional message that men shouldn't seem weak by asking for help. So, he accepted his depression as part of his character. He admitted that Covid intensified his depression, as he worried for the health of himself, his fiancé, their nine-year-old son, and his friends. He says he wished he had not brushed off his earlier need for help and has since become a proponent of therapy.

Democratic Senator John Fetterman admitted to having "dark conversations" about harming himself until he sought treatment. He worried that news about his treatment would end his political career. He didn't know what the outcome would be until he left Walter Reed at the end of March 2023, after six weeks of inpatient treatment with his condition "in remission."

Always seeming happy to everyone around him, comedian Howie Mandel also admitted to depression. He says it's challenging when he's alone. He finds that his standup routines distract him from the voices in his head. The Mayo Clinic describes the intrusive, unwanted thoughts that can manifest as phobias, compulsions, and anxiety. Mandel told Joe Rogan, "I feel like I'm balancing on this little ledge all the time." Comedy, exercise, and medication are his saviors.

The 29-year-old stud with all the famous and gorgeous female celebrities hanging on his arm, Pete Davidson, seems to have everything any dude could want. But he also suffers from depression. "I'm always depressed, all the time. I have to bring myself out of it constantly. I wake up depressed," he revealed. He toys with the psychedelic ketamine and went to rehab to withdraw from some of the drugs he was taking to squash his depressed state. Yet, the beloved "Friends" star Matthew Perry died from the acute effects of ketamine, so that may not be a safe solution.

Psychiatrist Sam Grazer, who treats Wall Street traders, investment bankers, and corporate attorneys, says there has been a surge in drugs, alcohol, and depression since the pandemic. People seeking help flock to legal ketamine therapy that provides an IV drip of the hallucinogenic drug that costs $750 per session. Elon Musk admits to microdosing ketamine to handle his depression. Silicon Valley executives have been regularly engaging in psychedelics to boost their business edge, The Wall Street Journal reports.

The recipients of ketamine are especially concerned about keeping their habit on the down low because clients want their big-ticket money manager to be on top of his game. Depression in the financial sphere has become such an issue that big banks like JPMorgan have created initiatives to deal with employees' mental health. However, other financial companies still ignore this need.

Male depression is often unrecognizable because it looks different from female depression. Men have eating disorders that no one can see (ignoring their high blood sugar or high blood pressure), erectile dysfunction that remains inside their pants (self-medicating with male performance aids), fatigue, sadness camouflaged by the more acceptable rage and anger, the inability to perform daily chores, increasing irritability, lack of concentration, relationship issues at work and home, sleeplessness, boozing and drugging, and having suicidal thoughts.

Sometimes, even family members are unaware of the demons living inside a relative's soul. The American Psychological Association warns that men's mental health is tested when a once-loving union is challenged. Too many men going through breakups deem themselves failures because their seeming virility could not sustain love. Most men I know leave a relationship without knowing what happened and why. They think it's "soft" to probe unanswered questions. However, if this work is not done, depression will ensue, and the same issues will repeat themselves in the next relationship.

Two-time PGA Tour winner Grayson Murray, living in Florida with his fiancé, committed suicide at the young age of 30. He had a close family, a love interest, and a bright future. It made little sense to anyone. He had previously talked about battling depression and alcoholism. After winning the Sony Open in January 2024, Murray admitted to being sober for eight months. And he said that life was "so good" for him then. "I wouldn't trade anything. I have a beautiful fiancé. I have beautiful parents. I have beautiful nephews and siblings."

He lovingly credited those close to him who had been through the struggles with him, calling it a "team effort." In a tribute, his caddie said, "He would truly do anything for anyone." That may have been the problem; he didn't save space to do enough for himself.

In January 2022, Dale L. Cheney, 46, with everything to live for, plunged off a New York rooftop. He was a dad of three, a financier with a Harvard MBA, he lived in a sprawling six-bedroom, seven-bathroom home worth nearly $4 million, and held board memberships and investments at six companies in four states. After a domestic dispute with his wife, she filed a restraining order against him. It was only one day before he jumped that he filed for divorce.

What caused the financier to commit suicide will never be fully understood. But a man's family bond that is suddenly broken is an excellent place to begin asking questions. Men are more dependent on their relationships than most people know. But unlike women who freely gab with their girlfriends, men are conditioned to conceal their pain.

Lately, the news has been peppered with stories of men committing murder/suicides against themselves and their innocent families. In Phoenix, Arizona, on Christmas Eve, three people were found dead. The shooter was identified as David De Nitto, 47, the widower of Maricopa County attorney Allister Adel, the first woman to hold this office. I spoke to this couple at many community events, and they seemed like an average, hard-working family. Allister served from 2019 to 2022, and it was her job to decide if and how people were investigated and charged with crimes. She resigned in March

2022 amid controversy over her fitness to fulfill her duties. She had undergone two brain surgeries to treat a blood clot, then spent time at a rehab facility for anxiety, eating disorders, and alcohol abuse.

A month after she left office, she died at age 45 of "health complications." Now, only a year later, her quiet financial advisor husband had an altercation with the woman he was seeing, and then used the gun on himself and her mother. Two young sons are now left orphaned. Quiet, unassuming men who have not processed grief are ripe for blowing a gasket. Concealing pain until a gasket is blown mimics Will Smith's famous Slap.

On the morning of the day after Christmas, 2023, 56-year-old Tom Cooper, remembered as a "lovely, lovely man," jumped to his death from his apartment building on New York's elegant Upper East Side. A co-worker described him as "extremely professional, genuine, and very kind." He had recently helped close an $18.5 million six-story townhouse and excitedly posted about it on Instagram. His clientele consisted of high-end people with high-end properties. He left a suicide note.

The most significant increases in suicides in the United States exist in older adults. Deaths rose nearly seven percent in people aged 45 to 64 and more than eight percent in people 65 and older. The CDC said that white men, in particular, have very high suicide rates.

Billionaire Thomas H. Lee, 78, once known as "the envy of Wall Street," shockingly committed suicide at his Manhattan,

New York office. He had built his fortune in the leveraged buyout industry. As a philanthropist, the married father of five and grandfather of two supported various charitable causes. He was so well-connected on both sides of the political aisle that the Democrat Clintons and the Republican Dr. Oz attended his funeral. With everything that seemed to be going for him, the question remained: "Why would he end his life?" His own family remained clueless. His brother's eulogy insightfully said, "There's a lot about each other we don't know. We want everybody to think everything is okay all the time. We owe it to Tom, and we owe it to ourselves to talk to each other and not hide behind walls. Tom, you were the master of the universe." Sadly, "masters of the universe" are not always as they seem.

The 1897 poem "Richard Cory" by Edward Arlington Robinson proves that a display of splendor doesn't always reflect what's in a psyche:

> "And he was rich—yes, richer than a king—
> And admirably schooled in every grace:
> In fine, we thought that he was everything
> To make us wish that we were in his place . . ."

The poem shockingly concludes with:

> "And Richard Cory, one calm summer night,
> Went home and put a bullet through his head."

There is often pent-up pain hiding in the psyches of men trying to play at being stoic.

PART III

10 WAYS HETERO MEN HIDE

Everything in life boils down to two questions: "How much?" and "How soon?" Relationships rule our world. And each one is set according to how much closeness we want and when it should begin.

Sun Tzu
"Victorious warriors win first and then go to war, while defeated warriors go to war first and then seek to win."

Winning first involves calculating strategies that assure success before any action is taken.

Sun Tzu
"The general who wins a battle makes many calculations in his temple before the battle is fought."

I remember meeting a blind date with whom I felt no connection. We went to dinner and had not even started the salad when this guy asked, "Do you sleep with a guy on the first date?" My sexual strategies were not going to become a pop quiz. As politely as possible, I responded that I must feel connected with someone for me to get physical, and that takes time.

As though he hadn't heard me, Blind Date pushed, "How long before you sleep with a guy?"

I courteously responded again, "Each situation is different."

Blind Date pushed harder, "Well, give me an approximate date. Weeks or Months?"

Not only wasn't I into him, but I was also fed up with his rude pressing. I said, "Ok, take out your calendar."

While this was tongue-in-cheek for me, he actually complied! I chose 17 months later and said, "That seems like a good date. Mark it on your calendar."

I rose from my chair and left the table. My "How much?"/"How soon?" tolerance had expired.

* * *

It was early in Tom's relationship with Alice, and their chemistry was off the charts. They were at different stages in life, but they were both kinesthetics who craved the sensation of touch, especially each other's. Alice asked him, "What are two kinesthetics to do?" He responded with no better word than "intertwine." So, the pair deliciously intertwined. Tom was more relaxed than Alice had ever seen him. But he abruptly stopped and declared, "It's too soon for us to have sex," as though they had just been embroidering for the past heated hour. He continued, "We've only seen each other two times." He did not mention the myriad hours they spent texting and phoning. This guy processed information visually, and only face-to-face contact computed for him. Tom was a left-brain accountant moved by math, while Alice was a right-brain social worker stirred by emotion.

Many factors enter into the "How much?"/"How soon?" question. They include people's backgrounds, their modalities for processing information through visual, auditory, or kinesthetic/feelings channels, how emotionally available they are, their relationship goals, and how safe they feel.

Unbeknownst to him, Tom was doing Alice a favor by initiating the "Let's hold off on 'having sex'" conversation according to his definition. She had no intention of going beyond where they were because when a man's Flap A penetrates a woman's Slot B, an emotionally deeper connection occurs. Tom said that if he didn't call Alice for a few weeks (obviously relaying a pre-meditated escape), he didn't want to hurt her. He already knew that doing the deed would come with expectations he would not fulfill—like calling regularly, being emotionally available, and becoming partner-dependable. Tom was confirming his emotional unreliability. Alice told him he needed to decide what he wanted before involving her. They never spoke again.

Gynecologist Christiane Northrup explains, "The cervix of a woman is at the top of the vagina. It is the reflexology zone of the heart." Intercourse stimulates the heart through the vagina by increasing prolactin and beta endorphin levels. As a woman's vulnerable area, cervical stimulation could incite a woman's addiction to a lover. Therefore, despite an urge to merge, until a couple agrees on social and sexual boundaries, it's wiser to wait. How long? That's the "How much?"/"How soon?" quandary singles face in this hurry-up-and-do-it-now culture.

The SAGE Journal of Social and Personal Relationships found that men will fall in love 69 days into a union, while women don't consider it until 77 days later. Therefore, the 3-Month Dating Rule for waiting for commitment is a good idea. Besides, that's when the honeymoon period wears off, and the real person begins to emerge. The "I love you" confessional occurs after 107 days for men and 122 days for women.

One dating website asks what a person wants. Some men check "something casual," others check "friendship," others check "sex," still others check "a relationship," but, surprisingly, many people check "I don't know yet." If a man doesn't know what he wants, why is he on a dating site? How will he know if he finds "it" if he doesn't know what "it" is? An "I-don't-know-yet" response is reason enough to swipe left.

Marrieds, too, should understand the "How much?"/"How soon?" dogma to sustain their union. Cara and Mark were traveling to the Bahamas on their first vacation. They had been married for two years, and they'd each been working much too hard. Going on frequent business trips was a legitimate way for Mark to keep his coveted distance while in a committed marriage. Mark needed his space, a topic he had never discussed with his wife.

Settled onto the airplane for their trip, they found their three-across row. Cara was in the aisle, and Mark was in the middle. Since no one sat in the middle seat, Cara was shocked that Mark moved to the window, leaving the seat between them empty.

Opposites attract and make for a healthful matching of jigsaw puzzle pieces. Those people you once deemed not your type may change your life! Appreciating compatible jigsaw puzzle pieces is only possible if two people can discuss their differences without constraint. Most couples don't have a clue about these differences!

Propinquity or closeness is a topic few couples discuss. But it can be a powder keg if a romance hits a rough patch—and which romance doesn't? A relationship can't survive without respecting each other's boundaries and communication needs.

Men often believe they prove their love not by words but by sticking around. Most women want to hear the words.

Gilda-Gram
Everyone has a Propinquity Quotient (PQ).
What's yours? What's your mate's?

Propinquity Score

- On a scale of 1 to 5, how physically close do you like to get to your partner?
- On a scale of 1 to 5, how physically close does your partner like to get to you?
- How similar are your scores?

We inhabit a lopsided gender world! Women are usually defined by attachment and threatened by separation. Men are typically characterized by separation and threatened by attachment. Even within those parameters, however, some men and some women require more or less propinquity, depending on their backgrounds. Talking this out at the beginning trumps dueling it out at the end.

With such chaos in this world, both men and women understandably try to shield their emotions from being battered. Beautiful supermodel Christie Brinkley said during her divorce that she didn't know who her husband Peter Cook really was.

Stunning celebrities get lonely for love like the rest of the population, and often overlook damaged men who cannot give them what they need. Brinkley named Cook's $3,000-a-month Internet porn habit and his desire for swinger sites in her divorce filing. Not to mention his 18-year-old mistress/assistant, who he conveniently kept around to "assist" his sexual appetite.

Caught red-handed and about to lose Brinkley's powerful connections, Cook's excuse was that *Christie* made him do it! Only an immature dimwit would blame another person for his dysfunctions. As you read earlier, porn users are not impressed with live women, anyway, even if their wife is a ravishing siren. So, Cook's "the-devil-made-me-do-it" excuse was as good as "the-refrigerator-made-me-fat" defense.

In the same vein, Rita Hayworth starring in the movie "Gilda," the name of her sexy character, said, "Men go to bed with 'Gilda,' but they wake up with me." Mirrors get foggy in the heat of a bedroom moment. Hayworth was expressing how her suitors were fascinated by her screen character but not able to fathom there was an ordinary woman with hungers beneath the Hollywood mask. *Should I change my name?*

Before contemplating a merger, every partner should categorize his PQ needs. Four levels of propinquity exist:

1. Superficial: One person depends on the other as his drug with sex organs.

2. Companion: Shared activity with one person can be interchanged with any other person.

3. Friend: The person you're with precedes the activity you share.

4. Relationship: Each partner desires to make himself worthy of the other's love.

One partner may want to eat dinner at a particular restaurant where the eatery takes precedence. The other partner may just want to BE with his partner no matter where they eat. Instead of inquiring about a potential mate's zodiac sign, PQ needs should take center stage.

<u>Gilda-Gram</u>
If a partner's self-protection
trumps protecting *you*,
you need another partner.

Someone terrified of getting close will allow no relationship to penetrate him. One person might try to push past his protective barrier, but the effort would be wasted. Either two people mutually want closeness, at least somewhat similarly, or why bother?

But people DO bother because there's a push in this world for people to become coupled. Aloneness is often ridiculed. Between boyfriends, attending a big movie premiere by myself one night, an alleged friend snarked, "Dr. Gilda is a relationship expert. But she has no relationship." As though love relationships are the only relationships that exist! Some women attach to a penis to fit other's expectations, whereas emotionally stable women wait for the right fit.

Christine Embe wrote, "While the past 50 years have been revolutionary for women, there hasn't been a corresponding conversation about what role men should play in a changing world . . . Men find themselves lonely, depressed, anxious and directionless."

Heterosexual guys are often terrified they're being taken in by their sex drives and being set up as "sexponents" and walking wallets, only to have their hearts broken. Yes, men hurt, too. But here we go again, if they show pain, they're termed "wussies," and wussies are "woke," the other side of "toxic." Is it any wonder men morph into a mode of self-protection?

In this woke age, here are 10 Ways Hetero Men Hide from Intimacy with a Hetero Woman.

CHAPTER 9

Sex-Possessed

Men often efficiently protect their hearts by going for sex instead of relationships. It's a remarkable segmentation of a man's life when sex and love dwell in different residences. But men's preference for just sex is problematic because most women want relationships.

Dominic Matthew Johnson writes,

"You think you've seen her naked because she took her clothes off?
Tell me about her dreams.
Tell me what breaks her heart.
What is she passionate about, and what makes her cry?
Tell me about her childhood. Better yet, tell me one story about her that you're not in.
You've seen her skin, and you've touched her body.
But you still know as much about her as a book you once found but never got around to open."

The Sex-Possessed just want the body. And they remain lonely and single despite hollow pleas for commitment. Women want a guy who wants to know them.

After a casual second dinner date, when Maddy returned home, she found an email from Norman with a very unusual "questionnaire."

It did not begin with, "I had a good time with you tonight." There was not even an "I'm-looking-forward-to-seeing-you-again" salutation. Instead, there was this: "These scenarios are all different. Rate each from 1-10 based on how the idea of the scenario stimulates your interest. LOL."

Maddy saw a list of 28 entries with what she found to be disgusting sex acts. She hardly knew this guy. Maddy sought a committed relationship, but Norman wanted the hot kinkies! The single woman wasted no time returning online for a better match.

In the eighties and nineties, the gorgeous Italian Fabio, with his hard body, ripped abs, pulsating pecs, and a mane of blond tresses blowing in the wind, graced the covers of romance novels. At 6'3" and 225 pounds, this adonis made millions of women swoon. Everyone was breathless and happy, especially since women who read romance novels are reported to make love 74 percent more often with their partners than women who do not. Women want to be swept off to nirvana while feeling they are loved. That can happen fictitiously between the pages of a romance novel.

However, according to Publishers Weekly, the woke world

has changed women's tastes in men both on the covers and inside. The once virile Italian stallion type on romance novel covers is replaced with a soft, sensitive, caring, "squishy-centered" guy with cats.

Hallmark's actor Kevin McGarry has become the latest leading man on the romance novel covers. Among other roles, he plays Mountie Nathan Grant in the drama, "When Calls the Heart." His character keeps striking out in love. The 38-year-old is not squishy-centered but wears a costume of law enforcement (Many women adore men in uniform.) while sensitively raising his niece as his own child. Audiences never see him without his shirt.

Fabio responded that this is "a trend, and it will change. It's ridiculous, like all the rest of the woke movement. Many women tell me, 'We can't find Real Men anymore,' and 'We want a Real Man.' The new romance novels are detached from reality."

The questions posed to Fabio are the same questions I get: "Where are the Real Men?" Women seek Rambo, but instead they're landing Dumbo. I hear the famished cry for men with backbones. The women who speak to me are more discerning than they ever were, and they want GQ plus IQ plus EQ. They want a man who does not call out his own name during sex. They don't want guys with thighs thinner than their own. One woman revealed her marriage went south the moment her husband put on her earrings!

Despite Fabio's objections, new covers and storylines are

planned to feature sexy trans men as the male hero for the "chicks-with-dicks" crowd. A 30-year-old top romance novel editor said, "We're finding that the romance novel readership is a lot younger and more liberal and more open to the trans revolution that's happening in society." When asked by a reporter, the 30-year-old editor did not know who Fabio was. Is it possible that the Harlequin-type romance novels deliberately squashed older swooners to favor woke millennials?

Now in his 60s, Fabio's hunky romance novels and products continue to sell. Baby Boomer women long for the strong, silent type like Fabio. Millennials swoon for tattooed, soymilk sippers. Gen Z ladies prefer "golden retrievers," who, like their namesake dog breed suggests, are sweet, gentle, easily trainable, and eager to please. With each incarnation into another kind of man, masculinity as we've known it alters—and those in the past tense mourn.

So now men ask, "How masculine is too macho, and how mushy is too soft?" A man online moaned, "The world sees us Americans as pansies in a dress whose men can't make up their minds if they are men at all."

CHAPTER 10

Gender Bender

The question of masculinity and all its current-day permutations suddenly reached a fever pitch on April 1, 2023, when Dylan Mulvaney, 26, landed an endorsement deal with the official beer of blue-collar America. Storms erupted on both sides of the woke ocean when she shared a social media video with her 10.8 million TikTok followers and 1.7 million followers on Instagram. With such a broad reach, companies were ripe to use her as their pitchperson.

The video depicted a can of Bud Light with Mulvaney's face on it to commemorate her one-year coming-out celebration as transgender. Just two days later, conservative musician Kid Rock retaliated with his own video that depicted him shooting up cans of the beer with a semi-automatic rifle and yelling profanities about the parent company, Anheuser-Busch. Country music legend Travis Tritt joined the fray and refused to carry Bud Light on his tour. Calls for boycotts of the beer became rampant, and anti-trans backlash began to spread. The boycott also crushed other beer sales in the Anheuser-Busch portfolio, including Budweiser, Michelob Ultra, and Stella Artois.

To flame the fires, on April 5, Mulvaney announced a collaboration with Nike, posting an Instagram ad modeling a sports bra (for her flat masculine chest) with leggings. By April 6, conservative backlash against Mulvaney's Nike partnership rose, including from trans Olympic athlete Caitlyn Jenner. Mulvaney posted a TikTok response to Jenner, attracting more than 5 million likes, criticizing her for using her enormous platform to invalidate another transgender woman's identity.

Finally, on April 14, Anheuser-Busch CEO Brendan Whitworth was pushed to release an Instagram statement that the company "never intended to be part of a discussion that divides people. We are in the business of bringing people together over a beer." By not naming Mulvaney or the controversy, his message was deemed wimpy and mocked by both sides of the debacle.

By May, the Mexican lager Modelo Especial replaced Bud Light as America's top-selling beer, a title it held for over 20 years. Anheuser-Busch tried to compensate with a new 15-second ad ahead of the July 4th holiday weekend featuring Chiefs tight end Travis Kelce and macho men sitting in their backyards opening Bud Light cans while grunting. That compensatory ad flopped.

To compound their already-depleted image, PETA discovered that Budweiser had been using Clydesdale horses for years in its marketing campaigns. On July 18, PETA claimed the company "quietly severs the magnificent horses' tailbones" so the horses appear more powerful when hitched to a beer wagon. PETA sent a letter to Kid Rock asking him to stop serving the beer in his steakhouse in Nashville, Tennessee, as a protest against the cruel treatment of the animals. Although Kid Rock had shot through the Bud Light cans, he was spotted selling the beer in his restaurant. So, PETA added its voice to the fracas.

Finally, on July 27, the company announced it was laying off 400 workers at its corporate offices. Anheuser-Busch had already axed the two marketing executives involved in the Mulvaney campaign and the outside ad agency that hired her. Somehow, the CEO kept his job, which made observers wonder whether soft male executives are the preference for a new woke America.

On September 9, it was announced that Bud Light sales were down 30 percent six months after the Mulvaney disaster. Beer Business Daily publisher Harry Schuhmacher concluded these beer drinkers were "lost forever." He opined that it is likely the company will continue to see similar year-over-year declines for the "foreseeable future." He said, "It's worse than just lost sales because now it's becoming systemic within the industry, and they're losing the retailers' confidence, and that's when it starts getting bad. We've never seen anything like this in the beer industry." All because a Y chromosome chose to prance around as an X.

In September 2023, Bill Gates's Foundation Trust bought 1.7 million shares of Anheuser-Busch InBev. This purchase worth $96.59 million could have given the parent company of the formerly top-selling U.S. beer manufacturer a shot at recovery. However, by the end of December 2023, it was reported that the brand had not, and the overall distaste for beer in general continued.

A new ad for Budweiser involved men slapping each other in the face until one drops. This "Power Slap" is part of Anheuser-Busch's six-year $100 million branding partnership with Dana White, the CEO of UFC and a Power Slap champion. White appeals to the demo Mulvaney's presence lost—but do Power Slappers represent mainstream beer drinkers?

Still desperate to bring back their brand, Bud Light offered Sylvester Stallone a $100 million endorsement deal. Unlike Travis Kelce, Stallone barked, "I'm not saving your woke brand."

Researching his book, "Go Woke, Go Broke," Charles Gasparino found that Budweiser settled on the Mulvaney representation because of corporate DEI mandates demanding more diversity. I covered the financial aspect of the controversy in my National Enquirer column with the headline that said it all: "Bud Light Brew-Haha Is Just Business." Indeed, the Mulvaney trans marketing ploy was not about supporting the underrepresented, but increasing revenues.

Once America's most popular beer, Bud Light is now Number 3 and down a billion dollars. The pendulum swings from one extreme to another in all social situations until it finds its modicum. In this case, the pendulum swung from woke to a joke. Ultimately, Anheuser-Busch could not Power Slap its return to its core audience of hetero men.

Hercules Speaks

The man who played Hercules, Kevin Sorbo, took on the topic of gender-altering treatments for young children. He said, "Let kids be kids. Let them get older and decide for themselves. If they think they were born in the wrong body when they're older—that's none of my business. But to tell this to 3-year-olds, 4-year-olds, 5-year-olds, 6-year-olds—and to confuse them when they're kids is crazy to me."

Sorbo sarcastically posted: "So, 19-year-olds shouldn't have to pay student debt because they can't understand the student loans they sign. However, 4-year-olds can change gender whenever they feel like it. Got it."

Elon Musk revealed he was "essentially tricked into signing documents" for his child to be treated with puberty blockers. "Xavier" became "Vivian Jenna Wilson" while Musk was in the dark.

"I lost my son. They call it deadnaming because my son is dead. Xavier is dead, killed by the woke mind virus," Musk said. "I vowed to destroy the woke mind virus after that."

California's Governor Gavin Newsom signed a new student gender identity law that blocks parents from being notified about changes in their child's gender identity or sexual orientation without the child's permission. Musk called this "the final straw." He moved the headquarters of Space X and the social media site X to Texas.

Gay fitness guru Jillian Michaels took the same stand as Musk about forbidding kids to alter their gender before their brains can maturely decide. She moved to Florida when she heard that her home state of California forbade parents to even know about their minor children's gender transition.

A young woman who transitioned too soon from female to male and is sorry about this procedure is suing the American Academy of Pediatrics (AAP) because she "doesn't want this to happen to other vulnerable young girls." Isabel Ayala is the litigant in this first-of-a-kind case filed in Rhode Island. While other detransitioners have sued medical practitioners, this is the first case to target the AAP directly.

At age eight, Isabel began precocious puberty after she had been sexually molested as a child. She resented the femininity she blamed for her molestation, and she believed she would be better off as a male. With prompting from the Internet, Isabel came out as transgender at age 12, assuming the change would fix her. To acquire the transition drugs, she learned to fabricate suicidal ideation and thus manipulated doctors and her family to support her while she threatened to kill herself.

Dr. Jason Rafferty, chair of the American Academy of Pediatrics' LGBTQ+ Health and Wellness Committee, put her on testosterone to treat her gender dysphoria, anxiety, depression, PTSD, and suicidality after only one hour-long visit. His AAP guidance is touted as the standard of care for physicians treating trans youth nationwide. No psychosocial analysis was done, and there was no mention of Ayala's previous diagnoses of autism, ADHD, and PTSD. Less than a year later, the young woman unsuccessfully attempted suicide.

At 17, after recognizing her transition had been a big mistake, Ayala decided to present as a female again. At 20, she suffers from unwanted body hair, Hashimoto's disease, vaginal atrophy, and bone alterations. Her story is the subject of a documentary produced by the Independent Women's Forum's "Identity Crisis" series.

Many schools encourage young people in crisis to decide their sexual fate independently of their parents. On a cross-country overnight trip to Philadelphia and Washington, D.C., a Colorado school district assigned an 11-year-old fifth-grade girl to share a bed with a biological boy who identifies as transgender. This arrangement lacked parental knowledge or consent. The boy's parents said he was in "stealth mode," where students were not supposed to know he was a boy.

It was the boy himself who revealed his identity. The girl he shared a bed with snuck into a bathroom to call her mom, fearing social backlash from classmates for requesting a different room. Kate Anderson, director of the Center for Parental Rights at Alliance Defending Freedom, said, "This practice renders it impossible for parents to make informed decisions."

The boy was moved to a different room, but nobody knew why. The school district had assured parents that boys and girls would be housed on different floors. The complaint claimed the trans-identifying boy's "privacy and feelings were always the primary concern," not considering the effect on the other students. Parents are losing clout over their children's welfare.

* * *

Sorbo attacks TV sitcoms for painting Dad as a chunky, out-of-shape, ineffectual fool while Mom's a hot chick on the make. The teen kids ridicule and dishonor their father, thereby crushing patriarchy and the nuclear family.

A university dean I know shared that his 16-year-old daughter came home from school one day and told him he was a "toxic male." He was devastated. Where did this come from? He had earned a Ph.D. and a J.D. by age 30. He had been highly educated in Christian schools and universities. He moved his family to fine communities to provide his kids with the best educational resources. Now this?

Sorbo says the sitcoms demean the biblical ideal that honors the father and the mother. He disavows Hollywood's anti-man campaign that has been portraying men as weak. His contrarian projects celebrate family, faith, country, and freedom—and now with his children's book, masculinity. He moved out of L.A.

* * *

The Bud Light controversy made the word "transsexual" a more commonplace concept. Its issues have now moved into schools. In 2023, a Missouri high school suffered backlash for making a transsexual student Homecoming Queen. Naming a non-female "Queen" was not a new custom for the school; it had done the same thing in 2015. The school said it was the students themselves who voted for these choices. Anti-LBGTQ+ groups targeted the new queendom, including Riley Gaines, the former college swimmer who criticized the NCAA for allowing the trans swimmer Lia Thomas to compete against her.

At Roanoke College in Virginia, a trans student wanted to join the women's swim team. The women knew the trans person before the transition and were supportive of his choice to do as he wished. But they drew the line when he competed against them because he had a biological edge.

Mirroring the Lia Thomas debacle, the issue began to tear the team apart. With all the controversy, the trans swimmer said she felt suicidal. Her compassionate swim teammates were stressed and angry and did not know how to handle this. The trans withdrew from the team. In October 2023, Lia Thomas bowed out of competitive swimming because of *"the constant battle to seek acceptance."* She finally conceded, "Nobody wants me on their team."

A meme on the Internet said, "Calling all mediocre males! Women's medals, records, scholarships, and sponsorships are now up for grabs! Live your dream by ruining theirs." The issue also punctuated the world's 2024 Olympics.

Tennis legend Martina Navratilova criticized the cyclists. Piers Morgan questioned why more women were "not standing up against this assault on their rights." Podcaster Megyn Kelly called this situation "infuriating," and former NCAA swimmer Riley Gaines offered to pay female cyclists to boycott future USA Cycling competitions.

However, Democrat Representative Alexandria Ocasio-Cortez from New York argued that if biological men are barred from women's sports, all underage women will face "genital examinations." *Really?*

The rage from families over this issue is palpable. An angry man online posted, "I don't believe that men who 'feel' like they should've been women should be able to use restrooms or showers designated for biologically authentic women. If one of those guys does try to use a restroom that my granddaughter is in, I will personally rearrange his plumbing, so he really is more like a woman than a man."

Thirty-year-old Justine Lindsay became the first openly transgender NFL cheerleader. Elle Magazine called her "an agent for change from within the macho-est of macho sports." Yet, she describes the difficulties of starting a new chapter for NFL cheer while coping with social media bullies and intolerant football fans.

The upset towards the trans community continues. In 2022, an Indiana high school crowned a drag queen as prom king. A year before, an Ohio high school crowned a lesbian couple Prom King and Queen. While parents may reject these crownings, their children have already gotten used to the trend and are voting against tradition.

Saint Mary's College in Notre Dame, Indiana, announced it will allow biological males to attend the all-women university if they have a history of identifying as women. But Pope Francis had said, "Gender ideology today is one of the most dangerous ideological colonizations." Yet, right before Christmas 2023, the Pope announced that the Church will now bless people in same-sex *relationships,* but not *same-sex marriages,* which the Church continues to oppose. Confusion abounds.

After the announcement of the inclusion of biological men in their dorms, the fur at St. Mary's went flying. One student posted, "It is no longer a women's institution. This is fraudulent misrepresentation at best. They have abandoned their faith, and they've abandoned the women. No woman should be forced to share a bathroom or living quarters with a man." Nonetheless, St. Mary's began accepting transgender applicants in the fall of 2024.

* * *

Beyond the walls of the divided schools, the world also began to see brands taking sides. Just as one side of the woke ocean had a list of "Best Places to Work for LGBTQ+ Equality," the other side created a "Refuse to Buy" register!

Target rolled out its "PRIDE" collection featuring LGBTQ-friendly clothing for kids, with "tuck-friendly" construction and extra-crotch coverage. The company lost $9 billion in market value when angry consumers called for a boycott of the retailer. The American Conservative Values ETF divested its holdings in Target.

Target CEO Brian Cornell defended the LBGTQ-friendly merchandise as "the right thing for society." However, "society" rebelled with threats to workers and damage to merchandise, prompting Target to remove some "Pride Month" items from its stores. Conservative commentator Tomi Lahren warned that Target "was about to get Bud Lighted."

By 2024, the Target Pride collection was back after the hoopla but had shrunk from 2000 items to just 75, down 96 percent. To further save its bottom line, the retailer's Pride selections were less flamboyant and limited to only certain stores.

However, earnings soared when Abercrombie & Fitch relaunched their brand to play to millennials and the younger Gen Z consumers. They expanded into curvy, gender-neutral, and Pride collections while partnering with The Trevor Project that advocates for suicide prevention and crisis intervention for LGBTQ+ youth.

Abercrombie took heat in the past for their superior attitude: "We go after the cool kids, the attractive all-American kid with a great attitude and a lot of friends. Many people don't belong in our clothes, and they can't belong. Are we exclusionary? Absolutely."

It's different now. Abercrombie is reaching their audience by partnering with advocacy causes.

The military also suffered a gender debacle. Drag queen Harpy Daniels was an active duty sailor in the Navy when they asked him to be its "digital ambassador," one of five such positions. The Navy hoped it would increase diversity. Rep. Jim Banks (R-Ind.) was told the program did not exist when in reality it did. Banks steamed, "We are facing a historic recruitment crisis, and instead of focusing efforts on strengthening our force, the Biden administration is forcing wokeness on our service members." Concerned about preparedness to defend our country, lawmakers said, "Promoting drag shows does nothing to enhance military readiness and war-fighting capabilities."

The epitome of confusion occurred with Alabama Mayor and pastor F.L. "Bubba" Copeland, a married father of three and local grocery owner. He was outed as having a secret life as transgender "Curvy Girl." He allegedly used a photo of a minor to encourage kids to transition. He also wrote erotic slasher fiction using the real names of women in his small town of Smiths Station, prompted by watching women on security footage from his store. He described murdering a woman in his community and used her real name.

When his unlikely story made the news, authorities conducted a welfare check on the mayor. While driving on a county road, police flashed their emergency lights, and he got out of his car and shot himself!

LGBTQ+ people are expanding their numbers. Like all social movements, their acceptance will be fraught with uncertainty and anger before peaceful resolutions are devised. Some corporations are catering to these gender benders not because they're in sync with the cause, but because they believe it's good for their bottom line. For young people, being accepted rules their goals. Adults can do as they please. But young, confused brains not mature enough to make important life decisions may be taken in and manipulated by ad campaigns that don't care about them. Outspoken parents like Elon Musk and Jillian Michaels are taking a stand. Will others follow?

CHAPTER 11

Human Dropout

Men are finding myriad other ways to self-protect from intimacy. A Japanese man with an unknown identity decided to chuck the whole human race altogether and become a dog. The man said he wanted to be a dog since he was a young boy. Now he's spent six months and $14,000 to have someone design a life-size custom-made collie costume.

Not only are collies his favorite breed, but their size makes them accommodating for a human to kneel inside the fur. Moreover, the breed's long hair can conceal the human form. He calls the dog Toco, and he produces videos of his life as a dog. He uses his paw to wave to people, rolls over, plays fetch, pretends to eat dog food, and greets other dogs. Do other dogs know he's an impostor? One internet critic said, "Don't let this guy get close to your leg!!"

Like other men uncertain about their identity, Toco told the New York Post, "My desire to be an animal is like a desire to transform, a desire to be something I am not." The man added that he wears the costume mostly at home, and his family accepts it. The video of his first walk went viral.

Toco's aspirations include becoming a movie star. His YouTube channel already has 50,000 subscribers. He also wants to find love—doggie style—with a woman who likes dressing up as a dog. Are there niche online dating sites that advertise these proclivities?

Toco admits it's "physically strenuous" to spend a day on all fours. But he says it's worth it because of the fun and excitement he derives from the experience.

A psychologist named Toco a "theriac"—someone who identifies with a non-human species. In contrast, a "furry" is a subculture where people dress up as dogs and other animals and may have sex with one another. The New York Post estimates there are 250,000 furries in the United States.

Dr. Elizabeth Fein, associate professor of psychology at Pittsburgh's Duquesne University, said, "Therians might believe they are a cat soul reincarnated into a human body. Some furries are therians, and some therians are furries, but they are two distinct groups."

The word "therian" is short for "therianthrope" and derives from the Greek words "ther" for "wild beast" and anthropos for "human being." In the past, people who identified as animals were isolated until online chat rooms emerged. Then, they formed groups of like-minded others. One Seattle therian who explains herself as a wolf in a human body says she growls, barks, and howls.

Cosplay, or dressing up in costume, is very popular in Japan. One man commissioned a full-size wolf costume to fulfill his childhood dream of being an animal. The outfit set him back $23,000, but he said that wearing it gives him power he doesn't feel in his everyday life.

Dr. Kathleen C. Gerbasi spent years studying the therian and furry community with the International Anthropomorphic Research Project (IARP). The professor of psychology at Niagara County Community College said that hiding one's authentic identity is burdensome. She describes how some therians and furries "put on human" to fit in.

Without suffering from Dissociative Identity Disorder (DID), living an inauthentic life will eventually be revealed. And the upshot will undoubtedly be humiliating and stressful.

Research by the IARP, which had similar findings from the University of California, found that most furries are younger than 25, white, and male. Half live with their parents, and most are politically liberal. Only one-third of furries identify as heterosexual, while 63 percent identify as bisexual or homosexual.

As part of Anthrocon 2023, over 10,000 furries gathered in Pittsburgh, Pennsylvania, for the world's largest anthropomorphic conventions. Bedecked as animal characters, they said they enjoyed gathering with like-minded people.

Departing from the usual demographics of young men, Jason "Mizuhiro Neko" is a 40-year-old IT worker from New Hampshire who identifies as a cat with wings. Mark Redshaw, "Harpo Barx," is a 47-year-old truck driver from New York State.

Some prefer to name their sexual identity with "I am not gay; my fursona is." So, they de-stigmatize their image and relinquish responsibility for taking a declarative sexual stand.

The IARP findings support other data showing that furries are no more likely to experience dysfunctional fantasy or delusion than non-furries. But Helen Clegg of the UK's University of Northampton finds that Therians have high levels of schizotypy, which manifest as unusual and disorganized thinking patterns and interpersonal difficulties. This condition may turn into schizophrenia and discomfort with social interactions and relationships.

One 22-year-old female preschool teacher in Salt Lake City, Utah, influences young minds by day and dresses up as a furry by night. As a sideline, she creates costumes for other furries and sells them for $1,200 each. Most furries complain about the discrimination lodged against them. A headline-making Michigan school denied putting a litter box in one of the bathrooms for kids identifying as furries.

There have been reports of United Kingdom schools allowing students to experiment with "neo-genders" and identify as non-human animals. Students in schools across

Britain have been allowed to identify as dinosaurs, horses, and moons.

With most therians and furries being adult men, hiding behind a costume dissociates them from the rigors and functions of manhood.

CHAPTER 12

Opportunist

Todd paraded false bravado as a lady's man with pecker power. He could pull off his rouse because he was tall, stately, and royally good-looking. Despite his being miserly, lonely wealthy women embraced his charms.

It was a freezing winter day, and Margo was heading to the Hamptons with Todd and his two kids, 7 and 9. The Hamptons is New York's tony summer playground on the Atlantic Ocean. It's a torturous bumper-to-bumper drive out of Manhattan's asphalt jungle every Friday night. But during the winter, when few Hamptonites visit their elegant homes, the traffic is less punishing.

True to chintzy form, Todd insisted on preserving the mileage on his ancient Jaguar. So, the foursome made the Hamptons trip in Margo's new Mercedes. She rationalized that the cheapness of her boyfriend of four months had little consequence since she made millions on her own.

With the kids typically squabbling in the back seat during the long trip, the group finally rolled onto Todd's gravel parking entrance in front of his sprawling stucco and glass estate. It was 10 pm when they arrived in the desolate darkness, amid a tooth-chattering 14 humid degrees.

Four tired bodies rushed to the front of this glass-enclosed house to get warm inside. Todd had shut off the electricity and hot water for the winter months. Margo and the kids asked him to turn on the juice immediately as they shivered in their heavy winter coats. He refused, saying he'd turn everything on in the morning. They were left to stumble into bedrooms in the dark, frigid house, arms outstretched as protection against bruising themselves on jutting furniture.

Margo tripped into one of the bathrooms to wash her hands and recoiled from the icy water. The outside cold had already numbed her fingers, so now the frigid water temperature made them feel frostbitten. She called to Todd again, pleading for warmth. But he stood firm against it.

Margo found her way into bed feeling not only dirty but angry, too. Todd jumped in beside her to cuddle. Furiously frozen, she would no longer accept Todd's frugality because she was in such discomfort.

Finally, morning came, and Todd turned on the water and the heat. He called his little daughter into the bathroom to give her a hot bath. After bathing the child, he called Margo to use the bathtub.

The woman slowly entered the hot bathroom with fogged mirrors.

"Yum! Warmth," she muttered.

But she gasped when she saw the child's dirty water still in the tub.

"Todd, you forgot to drain the water," Margo called.

Todd walked into the bathroom and calmly explained, "Honey, I didn't forget. You can use that same water for your own bath."

Margo panted, "The water is dirty—and now, cold."

Todd responded, "You can use it! She's only a little girl." In his beautiful, expansive glass-enclosed home in this wealthy community, this guy refused to shell out a few more coins for an additional tub of hot water.

Margo sighed, "Cheap with money, cheap with love." Todd's whiplash of his wallet-bearing wrist was his protection from intimacy. Plenty of other things were also missing. He flirted with women in her presence, although he swore he never put his penis in one—as though that was the only cheating factor of consequence! And he crassly suggested, "marrying you will be good for my business."

And she'd never forget the time she arrived at this Hamptons house when Todd ordered her to wash the massive glass windows in exchange for her "free weekend" away. He had already scheduled tennis games during that time, intending to leave her stranded as a domestic in the woods. He was shocked when Margo said she expected to be hosted, not ghosted. He innocently responded, "None of my other dates ever objected."

Couldn't he recognize that the last suit he'd ever wear would have no pockets? Sadly, nothing would buy this opportunist out of his emotional poverty.

That night, Margo escaped in her own car. She left skid marks.

* * *

Opportunists Abound

Margo returned to online dating for the first time in a long time. Most choices depicted a collection of lonely losers looking for a nurse and a purse in their sunset years. She spoke to a few nice guys, but each had quirks that raised flags.

One showed up in filthy jeans and heavy work boots. But his most unforgettable characteristic was the huge yellow pee stain on his fly. She left their coffee date gagging in mid-sentence.

Another was a tall, good-looking retired psychologist who had traveled the world. He wrote that he's "open to all possibilities. Please, no games. Love language is touching and eye-to-eye connection." Eye-to-eye? The guy wore dark glasses in all five of his photos! Swipe left.

Another advertised for an "attractive and personally

liberated woman for friendship, fun, No Strings Attached." He explained, "I am not seeking a committed relationship because I'm already in one."

There was a tall, dark, and handsome lawyer. When they met in person, he was 30 years older than his photo. She ran to the bathroom to vomit.

There was also a journalist who was beautiful in his photos. They exchanged texts, and they almost got to meet in person. However, Margo noted he never asked one question about her. She asked him why. He said he'd found out all he needed to know about her on Google. He was superficially happy to know *about* her, but chose not to know who she really was.

UGH! She was sick of the whole thing.

Then Barry popped up. She was intrigued by his extensive traveling, openness, intellect, and work in a cutting-edge industry. He was also 6'5" and BIG! When they met for coffee, his giant size made Margo feel protected.

On their second date, they hiked, lunched, and continued walking and talking under sunny skies. After a full and wonderful day, Barry drove her back to her house.

She enjoyed their intellectual palaver, and it was a perfect date. However, while sitting together in his car in front of her house, for no reason, he blurted out, "I'm frugal."

"Oh no!" she sighed. "Another Todd?"

In the dating world, each guy pays for the issues of the one before him. Because Margo had been with cheap Todd before meeting Barry, the mere mention of frugality rang warning bells.

He spoke about his world travels. Margo began to piece together his pattern. He would go online for dates before he traveled to a new country and procure a local woman. He'd live with her during his temporary stay to avoid paying rent. In support of her suppositions, he complained he was now staying with friends and had to sleep on the couch. Margo was supposed to say, "Oh, poor thing. Stay with me." But she was on to him.

She mused, "He calls himself *only* 'frugal'? 'Pimp' seems more fitting.

She was anxious to see what the lothario's next step would be.

They enjoyed a great day outdoors and concluded that they liked each other. Big Barry capped the tender moment with, "Why don't you invite me up to your place . . . so we can cuddle?"

Women know that "cuddle" is guy code for "f--k." Margo sensed she was being set up as this "frugal" pimp's next mark.

He had mistaken her for a welcome mat. She calmly explained to Big Barry that they hardly knew each other and it was too soon to become intimate on any level. As big as he was, he reverted into the Hulk in a sulk! Women observe how a man handles rejection: is it as a baby or as a grownup with grace? Margo had no intention of providing diaper service to this thumb-sucker. She let herself out of the car, and Barry was dust.

Some guys' attempts at self-protection will be tested when their potential prey audaciously and assertively questions, "What's in it for me?"

Margo began to feel sorry for herself for attracting such losers. Then she read that Kelly Clarkson had won a lawsuit for $2.6 million against her ex-husband, Brandon Blackstock, the father of her two children. He had overstepped his managerial role in her career and unlawfully procured deals that Clarkson's talent agent should have negotiated. One would assume a husband of seven years would have the best interests of his wife. Blackstock tried to overmanage his wife's career—and now he was court-ordered to pay her back the money.

Opportunists may be run-of-the-mill guys like Barry or big Hollywood players who narcissistically con top-earning wives under the guise of love. Opportunism is just another way heterosexual men hide from giving and loving.

CHAPTER 13

Credentials Extender

Men uncomfortable with themselves exaggerate their worth with an emboldened identity and distended credentials. The Dunning–Kruger effect describes people who assess their cognitive ability as more significant than it is. Whether distortion of the truth is intentional doesn't matter to an unaware recipient of their lies.

Naomi

One attractive-looking California man, Evan, with steel grey hair, chatted up Naomi on a professional business site on a lonely holiday weekend. His profile said he was a "self-employed construction engineer/project manager" with a Ph.D. The accompanying photos of his alleged work were gorgeous, and Naomi was impressed.

Having a Ph.D. herself, Naomi had met some architects in her time, but none boasted this advanced degree. She was curious why he felt that credentialing was necessary for his line of work. Evan and she began writing back and forth.

They chatted about past marriages and children and bantered about the political unrest in the world. Their diatribe seemed robust and quick, as Naomi liked.

At this point, not trusting anything guys wrote on their profiles, whether on a dating or professional site, the woman asked, "Do you really have a Ph.D.?"

Evan said, "Yep. I have a Ph.D. in civil engineering. I always wanted a Ph.D., and I got it. Having this degree at work is very important. Also, I have my B.S. in civil engineering."

It made no sense to Naomi, so she wanted to learn more. As though she had not heard him, she pressed, "What did you say your doctorate was in?"

He responded, "I'm a bit lost here, LOL! I ain't got no doctorate degree."

Naomi questioned, "You have a Ph.D.? Then why don't you call yourself 'doctor'?"

Evan said, "I do have one! As a Ph.D. holder, I'm qualified to be called Dr.?"

Naomi shot back, "Yes, it's a doctorate."

He said, "Yep. That's right. I have my Ph.D. in civil engineering."

Naomi said, "I was engaged to a civil engineer. He was skilled at stuff I couldn't even fathom."

Evan said, "OK. LOL."

Naomi was becoming bored with all these LOLs! Does this

guy even have an IQ? He changed the subject to, "Are you married?"

The attractive woman was baffled. How does someone go through the rigors of a Ph.D. program and not know he's entitled to be called "doctor"? How does someone with a Ph.D. say, "I ain't got no doctorate degree"? Something was fishy.

They discussed marriage, kids, past relationships, and more personal information. In describing his marriage, he defended, "The fault wasn't from me, but from my ex-wife. I had to stick with her, but in the end, she betrayed me. It's all life experience, though. What happened with your last relationship?"

Naomi explained some of the superficials. He fished, "Are you ready to date someone new soon?"

She answered, "Sure, if I meet someone I feel compatible with. I'm just unwilling to put up with lies and BS."

He said, "I agree. Why don't we continue communicating on WhatsApp?"

Naomi responded, "Let's speak on the phone first."

He responded, "Sure," and disappeared.

Naomi figured he probably knew she saw through his "lies and BS." The next day, she noticed he rechecked her profile. But as they say on the ranch, "big hat, no cattle"!

* * *

Elizabeth and Brenda were Ph.D. research scientists who worked for a large pharmaceutical company. Elizabeth knew

Brenda and her cardiologist husband were avid hikers, so she asked her work buddy to recommend a good mountain to hike for her second date with Charley. Charley was a tech genius who dropped out of college, Steve Jobs style.

When Elizabeth and Charley reached the recommended mountain, they were surprised to run into Brenda and her husband. The four of them had some friendly chit-chat for about 15 minutes. Elizabeth joked that this was now officially a mountain of doctors. The group laughed. That should have been the end of the observation. But feeling uncomfortable among the highly pedigreed threesome, Charley piped up that sometimes people call him "doctor," too. He was a college dropout! The other three hikers glared at him. Charley's insecurities were too apparent to miss.

Brenda and her husband detoured, and Elizabeth and Charley started their descent. As they walked and chatted, Elizabeth picked up other insecurities this man had. How could she date a man who needed to bolster his credentials to be in her company? That was the last time they saw each other.

Gilda-Gram
Intimacy is impossible with liars.

CHAPTER 14

Forked Tongue Wordsmith

When someone "speaks with a forked tongue," it signifies they say one thing while meaning or doing another. Usually, the person is deliberately duplicitous. If that person is a capable wordsmith, whether his platform is brief texts, lengthy emails, or face-to-face chatter, he will adroitly pull off his caper with the help of any recipient who wants to believe him. This game is especially prevalent with today's online interaction and media coverage.

South Carolina congressman Jeff Duncan, a self-described "life-long social conservative," campaigned to advocate for traditional family values and protect the nuclear family. At the same time, he was consorting in affairs during his 34-year marriage. His divorcing wife said his dalliances seemed to be an open secret around the political circles in South Carolina and Washington, DC. He scripted the rumor that his marriage had been loveless to justify his misdeeds. Then, he abandoned his entire family to live with his mistress.

How did voters feel about reelecting him? Based on his signature barbeque in August 2023 that grew from 400 must-attend conservatives to 2000, the world seems numb to another forked tongue wordsmith in the news.

Duncan is not the only truth-challenged politician whose dalliances haven't affected his political future. San Francisco's Democrat Mayor at the time, Gavin Newsom, entered rehab after apologizing for his affair with Ruby Rippey-Tourk, the wife of his deputy chief of staff, Alex Tourk. At the time of the affair, Newsom was in the process of divorcing his wife, then Fox News host Kimberly Guilfoyle, now engaged to Republican Donald Trump, Jr. Voters didn't care. Newsom was elected California's Democrat governor!

After 17 years of marriage and three children, Republican New York Representative Vito Fossella had a love child, told his mistress he was separated, and proceeded to fake two separate lives with both women. After the tabloids got hold of the congressman's cheating story, both his wife and mistress raged. A source said his wife knew he had a roving zipper, but she didn't think he had another child. *Huh?*

Describing the condom-less conundrum, reporter Andrea Peyser in the New York Post prescribed decades of therapy for their four humiliated kids. How did voters react? Since 2008, when Fossella's affair was all the talk, he continued to rise in the ranks of the New York Republican party. He became the Borough President of Staten Island! He and his wife are still married, and his baby mama is a Christian life coach.

Forked tongue wordsmiths wipe out tons of toner cartridges as they pump up their enticement. Do you think a guy can "logic" a woman into bed with words? Mirroring Cyrano de Bergerac, today's conversational booty camp is thriving because of our online interaction. With this trend, skillful writers and speakers are in their most fruitful element.

The 1897 story of Cyrano de Bergerac depicts an ugly, large-nosed man who feels unworthy of winning the love of Roxane. So, he writes her love letters signed by his handsome friend, Christian, who ultimately wins Roxane's hand in marriage. Thus, a man *can* seduce a woman with words—even if they're someone else's.

Christian dies in battle. While Roxane mourns his loss, in the throes of death himself and in Roxane's arms, Cyrano admits his wordsmithing. Roxane reveals she's known for a while that he wrote the letters, and she says she shares his feelings. His final line is about loving his pride more than ever loving Roxane.

Hetero men today have told me they feel safest when texting because possible rejection would not smart as profoundly as it might on the phone or in person. Like Cyrano, if today's male loves his pride more than he can love a woman, he must ask himself, "What am I trying to protect?"

Comedian Bill Maher wisely advises men, "If you want to get with a woman, try this trick: Talk to her. In person. The phone ruined dating and porn ruined sex, and women have been left with men who don't know how to talk to a woman anymore."

So, a forked tongue wordsmith pushes calculated words, reducing the sender's inhibitions and seducing his receiver's thirst for love. Wordsmiths easily hide behind salacious syllables that camouflage their loneliness and feelings of unlovability. An able male hetero wordsmith knows he can win favor with his heartfelt prose and turn-on tongue—because his target is always a needy woman blind to the fact that the communicator's tongue is forked.

Sadly, forked tongue wordsmiths keeps hiding and their unsuspecting women keep getting hurt.

CHAPTER 15

Cradle Robber

The Honey/Money ratio prevails. A fictitious billboard might boast, "Weak Egos Get Bragging Rights." No matter how much wealth and fame they have, insecure aging men try to impress the world with a fertile young babe on their arm. "Let my buddies salivate!" they reason.

Guinness World Records recorded that the oldest father in the world was Australian Les Colley (1898-1998), who fathered his ninth child at age 92 with a Fijian woman he met through a dating organization.

In more recent times, WWE legend 70-year-old Hulk Hogan married his third wife, 45-year-old yoga instructor and accountant Skye Daily. Oak trees do not produce acorns until they are at least 50 years old. So, guys pursue young women sometimes without marrying them but procreate with them. Just the feeling of being fertile may boost some egos.

Eighty-year-old Robert De Niro fathered a child with martial arts pro Tiffany Chen, 45. During a court trial with his ex-assistant of eleven years, Graham Chase Robinson said De Niro regularly bragged to his staff about his girlfriend 30 years his junior and made lewd jokes about his Viagra prescription. So, the world heard why he paired with his baby mama and how he medically kept it up.

Australian Associate Professor Tim Moss said, "There's a misconception that male fertility lasts forever. Older men take longer to get their partners pregnant, and there's a link between a father's age when children are conceived and some neurodevelopmental problems in their children." So, sperm count and quality of the sperm do fall with age.

After the baby was born, De Niro described the parents' division of labor: he supports the mom and newborn (There's the money!), and she does the mommying (There's the honey!).

Similarly motivated by the same heat for a youthful bedmate, De Niro's good friend, Al Pacino, welcomed a fourth baby at age 83 with his 29-year-old partner, Noor Alfallah. He could not have known his lady friend long enough for trust to be established because Pacino learned of the pregnancy when the mother was already in her sixth month.

Pacino has "medical issues" that would have ordinarily prevented him from impregnating a woman. He was so shocked that he could be the father he insisted on a paternity test. Alfallah obliged, and it showed that the baby was indeed his.

This May-December relationship paid off: A judge ruled that Pacino will pay his girlfriend $30,000 monthly in child support after giving her $110,000 upfront, paying $13,000 for a night nurse, and additional medical expenses not covered by insurance. Also, he will make a $15,000 yearly deposit in an education fund for the little guy. While the mom has primary physical custody, the pair will assume joint legal custody.

Seventy-three-year-old rocker Mick Jagger welcomed a baby boy with 20-year-old ballerina Melanie Hamrick. Rolling Stones guitarist Ronnie Wood married Sally Humphreys in 2012, the owner of a theatre production company, 31 years his junior. Four years later, they welcomed twin daughters just before Wood's 69th birthday. The guitarist quit smoking after undergoing treatment for lung cancer in 2017 and has been sober since 2010.

Internet Wisdom
"For every stunning, smart babe of 70,
there is a bald, paunchy relic in yellow pants
making a fool of himself with a 22-year-old."

Older men are not giving up on expanding their progeny. As an attempted public service announcement, outspoken Chelsea Handler said she wanted to "protect the women of the world" from the epidemic of "horny old men" like Pacino, De Niro, Musk, and Baldwin—all who have a propensity for procreation. The comedian joshed, "Don't get me started on these four horny old men who have never met a broken condom they didn't like. Between the four of those guys, they have 32 children." And lots of disposed of exes.

Ninety-eight-year-old Dick Van Dyke and his 52-year-old wife, Arlene Silver, don't have children. He hired her as his makeup artist, and they were friends before they started living together in 2011. She gushes about his positivity and happiness and how he got her to sing. They consider their age gap irrelevant.

* * *

Yet, according to WebMD, 1/3 of *women* aged 40 - 69 wouldn't want these old geezers anyway because they prefer *younger* men of ten-plus years. Younger men say they appreciate a woman who knows who she is. And they like that they can never get away with telling a lie to an older woman because she can see through them!

That didn't work out for Tony Danza who is one year *older* than his 1970s sitcom "Taxi" co-star, Marilu Henner. He said their romance fizzled because of her remarkable memory. He admitted that she remembers everything and "it's not something you want." Henner was on The View with him and laughed. She has Highly Superior Autobiographical Memory or H-SAM, a rare ability to remember specific details from specific dates. Having H-SAM might be threatening to a man who can't remember the lies he tells.

The May-December love story of Mary Tyler Moore and Robert Levine always enthuses me. In 1982, Moore's mother had bronchitis, so her daughter called her regular doctor, who was unavailable. Dr. Robert Levine was covering for him and made the house call. Since he had seen Moore's mom for the second time and knew her condition, he told Moore, "Next time there's an emergency, just call me."

Moore asked, "Does acute loneliness count?" The good doctor responded, "Yes." They went on a dinner date within a few days, started spending weekends together, and were married a year later—for 33 years until Moore died at 80. Moore was 18 years the physician's senior. The unlikely pairing sounded like an unusual Hollywood script, but this devoted husband accompanied her to various projects to help monitor her Type 1 diabetes and drinking problem. Levine told People Magazine he considered it his role and privilege "to be her protector and care for her and hold her." Together, they became a force on the international board of directors of the Juvenile Diabetes Research Foundation.

This is no Hollywood BS. About ten years before her death, I was in the Admiral's Club waiting for a flight from LAX back to New York. I spotted a tall, unassuming man with black-rimmed glasses diligently carrying a clinking china cup and saucer with steaming hot coffee. He was headed to the comfy lounge chairs across the room. Something about him oozed that this was a loving gesture. Not recognizing him, I was intrigued enough to follow him at a distance. Waiting comfortably for her husband's return was Mary Tyler Moore. I saw this man's adoration for his woman, which silently influenced my choices for partnership in the following years since I, too, am diabetic and hoped to find a loving partner that caring.

Researcher Samantha Banbury said, "Research examining age-gap relationships is sparse, particularly on women who date younger men." So, the Sexual and Relationship Therapy journal published a study of a small sample of cougars with a mean age of 45. These older women offered anecdotal evidence that their sex lives sizzle. Yet, "society tends to view women who date younger men more critically than older men who date younger women," Banbury said.

Ask Joan Collins about that! At 90, she addressed the 32-year age gap with her fifth husband. She said, "It doesn't matter; I can wear him out!" She notes her high enthusiasm for life, which her husband shares. She described how they began as great friends, working together on a play and hanging out. They saw each other the following year and began exchanging love letters. Gradually, they realized they were very much in sync.

The age differential worked differently for Mariah Carey and her backup dancer boyfriend, Bryan Tanaka, who were together for seven years. When he turned 40, he wanted a family. Mariah, at 54, had already parented kids with Nick Cannon, which led to their split. Sofia Vergara and Joe Manganiello divorced because Manganiello at 47 wanted to start a family, but Vergara, 51, already had a 32-year-old son with her first husband, and she was ready for the next phase of life.

Thus, for an older woman and a younger man who still want a family, age discrepancies are not as easy to navigate as they are for older men with younger women. Child-rearing should be discussed before commitment.

It's unknown whether the Honey/Money ratio played a part in the pairings of Mary Tyler Moore, Joan Collins, or Mariah Carey, because these women all enjoyed greater wealth than their men. But no matter their ages, two people are in sync when the *voltage* of their intensity-for-life matches. Eighty-year-old Sara was a regular in her Tai Chi class. Sixty-nine-year-old Brad approached her and said, "I like your energy." They have since been a high-voltage item for two years. The electric voltage that two people mirror has nothing to do with age.

According to a global survey of over 26,800 Bumble members, 59 percent of women said they're open to dating a younger man. Bumble expects these cross-generational relationships, named "gen-blend" unions, to surge. Overall, 63 percent say that age isn't a defining factor. Despite what old codgers can "buy," braggadocio can't replace great synched voltage.

Sexual Apparatus at Any Age

Men and women are confused about what they want in a partner at every age—until the right person interrupts their fears. As we age, our sexual apparatus ages, too. The male sex hormone, testosterone, decreases and may create problems for men to get erections. So, how do these men perform in the bedroom to make that sperm swim? De Niro already admitted in court that he takes Viagra. In addition, a new rage on the market since 2016 is dissolvable penis enlargement shots made of hyaluronic acid. Its objective is to boost confidence and improve performance. Products are temporary as the body metabolizes them over time, and they're also reversible. While the procedure is meant to increase girth, recipients also boast an increase in length.

So, is an extra .25 to .3 inch increase per treatment worth it? A behemoth bulge can last about three years with maintenance. Demand for the shots is swelling even at the steep cost of $11,000 to $20,000 for a round of treatments, depending on the size desired. This business is undoubtedly expanding: A Dallas-based enhancement firm started in 2020 now has 16 franchises nationwide.

Are older A-list men partaking in this male equivalent to female breast enhancements? There seems to be an increased interest in expansion these days—of progeny and penises.

Forty-six-year-old tech mogul Bryan Johnson is trying to reverse aging in his penis by 15 years through "painful" acoustic shock therapy on his genitals. He spends $2 million yearly trying to fight off the inevitable. The shocks create microinjuries that the muscles rebuild. He claims to have already seen results in two months. To this, he also adds a strict diet and exercise program.

Might the new and improved pecker predilection exist because the U.S. came up as the 59th shortest in the world on penis size compared to 90 other countries? Published by World Data, the study went viral in June 2023. The New York Post said there is no way to rank penis size by country. So, how did the researchers get their data?

Jen Caudle, a female physician on TikTok, tried to shatter the myth that size matters: "The average flaccid penis is 3.6 inches, and the average erect penis is 5.17 inches. Size is usually unrelated to sexual pleasure. One viewer commented, "Like money, what matters is what you do with it!"

Discussing erectile issues fills men with so much angst that urologists, especially female ones, had to come up with a visual of a 4-point erection hardness score when asking men to describe their turgidity. Accompanied by a childlike cartoon, "1" is a marshmallow and signifies no erection at all, "2" is a peeled banana that won't be able to penetrate, "3" is a curved banana that will penetrate, but in a rickety way, and "4" is a perfect cucumber that porn stars boast about, and all men envy.

Using this system, men can more comfortably describe their issue as a number rather than as an embarrassing description. This approach seems like children who announce whether they did #1 or #2 in the toilet. Turgidity evaluations infantilize men even more, supporting their avoidance of grown-up manhood and its responsibilities.

Can we get an Amen in support of grown up men?

CHAPTER 16

Ghost

Ghosting has become a popular pastime among gutless men (and women) because disappearing lets them off the confronting hook as they cowardly exit.

Ghosting disrespects the feelings of the one in the dark. Withholding is a form of abuse, but ghosting is becoming a popular way for men in crisis to hide from healthy interactions.

Carolyn gave Liz's telephone number to a "great guy." Liz liked Carolyn a lot, and she trusted her judgment.

Weeks went by and Liz never heard from the guy. She told Carolyn, "OK. He's not interested in meeting someone new."

Great Guy sent Carolyn this text: "I am experiencing some personal struggles right now, and the timing of meeting someone is just not right for me currently. I am sure your friend is very nice and please let her know it was not because I "wasn't interested." I am just keeping to myself for a while socially. Thank you for your friendship."

Carolyn apologized to her friend with a comforting, "Maybe down the line."

Liz responded, "He seems like a sensitive man. Timing is crucial. Thanks for thinking of me, anyway."

Six months passed, and Liz had forgotten about the intended setup. Then Carolyn texted her, "That Great Guy I was going to set you up with six months ago is ready to get into the dating scene. He asked for your number again. I gave it to him, and he said he'd contact you later this week."

Liz wrote, "There's something to say about a guy who knows when he's ready for stuff. It will be interesting to talk to a man with some depth."

"Glad to help! He's a really Great Guy. You never know."

Great Guy did not call Liz on the phone. Instead, he texted, "Hi. I'm Carolyn's friend. She and I have been talking, and I thought I would reach out to you to say hello. I'm sorry it's in the middle of the dinner hour, but I'm just leaving work. I just wanted to introduce myself. I'm going to run out and get some exercise this evening, but I wanted to let you know I will be reaching out further either after exercise or later in the week. I hope to meet you if that is something you would like to do."

Liz was pleasantly surprised at Great Guy's courteousness. But with all his wordiness, she suspected he was nervous and insecure.

Three hours later, he wrote again, "I'm sorry the tennis went a little later than expected this evening. If it is OK, I will try to get hold of you tomorrow evening, but at an earlier hour."

Liz responded, "Hi. No problem. Carolyn told me to expect to hear from you. Tomorrow should be fine. Have a good night."

Great Guy wasted no time to respond, "Nice to meet you. Yes, Carolyn told me she was going to warn you! Have a good evening."

He sent a photo of himself with a warm smile. He captioned it, "That's what I look like. Instant dating site."

Liz wrote back, "Friendly smile! Warning heeded :).

He didn't contact her the following evening as he said he would. Nor the evening after that.

Liz thought, "Overpromiser and underperformer. Another character who extends the truth."

But it was game on! So, Liz reached out to him. "Hi. Where have you gone?"

He responded immediately, probably somewhat embarrassed, "I am here. Just a little busier at work than I had hoped."

Liz asked, "Is that a good thing for you?"

He answered, "It's just the way it is for me. There will always be unexpected emergencies, and I am on the front line regarding who gets called. It's a good thing, I guess."

Great Guy owned a tech think tank, so tech issues were constantly occurring.

Liz asked, "Are you living the life you want?"

"It depends on how deep a level we choose to analyze. I have two children. They are happy and healthy. I have a healthy new grandson. Oh, that is wonderful. I am fortunate. I was unhappy in my marriage for the last 32 years, and I got divorced at age 59. I essentially started over financially as far as assets are concerned. Let's just say that part of my life hasn't turned out how I thought it would."

He continued, "Everything is relative. I wish I had made a better choice of partner initially so that I still would be happy in my marriage, but I have two wonderful children, and I would not have them without selecting the wife I did. So that's just the way it goes. I wouldn't go back and change anything, I guess."

Liz said, "I chose wrong, too, in my former marriage. Life doesn't exactly turn out as we expect. But I think that's just part of the journey. And the real objective is to grow from each poor choice."

"I agree with you. I always go back to the line from Monty Python and the Holy Grail: "Choose wisely."

"I have a commitment tomorrow evening, but I am free Saturday afternoon, evening, and Sunday afternoon."

Liz chose, "Let's make it Saturday. I'm free all day."

They continued texting for over an hour. Takeaway remarks that Liz pulled from their exchanges were:

> **Great Guy:** "I know texting is difficult. It is safe, but it is a bizarre form of communication as there is a prolonged pause between each response. It is quite fascinating. And it's only proper that you take turns. It is improper to have too many texts in a row without a response."

Liz: It sounds like he needs the "safety" of texting. It also sounds like he's giving a lecture on texting. Stuffy? Anal? OCD?

When Liz said she had no drama in her life, Great Guy commented, "What a lovely concept, dating someone who is not attached to drama."

Liz: He admitted to attracting drama-filled relationships. Why? A commitment phobe attracts drama to keep his distance. Liz had been guilty of that herself, but she was drama-avoidant now.

Great Guy: "It would be nice to just hang out with you, and I wish we were neighbors right now."

Liz: Sounds like a homegrown, down-to-earth guy who's lonely to find someone on his wavelength. I like that.

Great Guy: "You are the kind of person I like talking to, I think."

Liz: How can he jump to that conclusion from just an hour's worth of texts? Does he know what he's *feeling*? Does he know how to *express and share those feelings*? That's the kind of person *I* like talking to.

Great Guy: "Well, I wish we knew each other better. And I wish we were hanging out comfortably, talking to each other, playing footsie. Maybe sometime in the future."

Liz: Hmmm. Footsie already? He's into touch. A kinesthetic, like me. I like that. What is he imagining about our interaction?

Great Guy: "I spend a tremendous amount of time alone. Because I'm not a bar/happy-hour/pick-up-women kind of guy."

Liz: That mirrors me and is perfect for my life. But is he a loner or a hibernator hiding for self-protection?

Great Guy: "You and I are on the same page."

Liz: Good. He feels our commonality and our obvious good connection.

Great Guy: "I am hoping that we become good friends because I would love to have somebody drama free who enjoys my company and doesn't live a million miles away. And to be honest, that I can hang out with."

Liz: He wants deep friendship, as do I.

Great Guy: "I hope we can hang out together. I hope we like each other enough to want to do that because you seem like a fascinating person.

Liz: Fascinating? Why?

Great Guy: "I like to please."

Liz: Red Flag: This could be a deal-breaker for me. People pleasers tell lies to be liked. They trade their authenticity for approval. Great Guy lied through an unhappy marriage for decades, so he's had extensive practice acting instead of living. Pleasers put compatibility before commitment to avoid conflict. CAUTION!!

Great Guy: "I am an old-fashioned guy. I like to pick you up, instead of meeting you someplace."

Liz: I like that.

Great Guy: "One more thing. If you ever can't sleep, you can always text me in the middle of the night. I am on call all the time. So, I am used to getting up at all hours. But I am more than happy to be available to the people important to me."

Liz: That's BS! People pleasing in full view. We just met—and not even in person. I couldn't yet be important to him—unless he's living in some altered delusional state.

The Date

Great Guy picked Liz up in his car at her front door. She liked his kind, warm looks. She hugged him hello because they had texted for hours, and she felt the rapport. He looked surprised. "Is he an uptight character?" Liz wondered. She got into this stranger's car with total trust because it wasn't a date from an online meet market. Great Guy came highly recommended.

Since she knew nothing about where he lived, he drove her to his neighborhood, about 20 minutes from her. He took her to a breakfast nook, and they talked and laughed and laughed and talked. Did that check the list for the kind of "hanging out" he was after? An average person laughs about 15 times a day. This couple was way over their quota, and it promoted bonding. They had shared values, common cultures, and similar outlooks about the world.

She was having so much fun that he was able to seduce her into downloading the data for each career move she made. He listened intently, and when a story diverted to another topic, Great Guy returned to Liz's previous download and asked what happened after the last story. It was fun and filled with laughter but also very clinical. While getting intel on Liz, he never shared his life, how he worked, how he spent his days, the history of his marriage and divorce, or his social interactions. He did not reveal himself, except with some throw-away sentences here and there. He seemed closed down.

Liz thought they would have the whole day and maybe the evening, as their original text exchange intimated. So, there was plenty of time for more in-depth talk. He repeated that he enjoyed good conversation and hanging out.

After about an hour of their merriment, Great Guy said he cannot sit still and "Let's go." Just like that! Liz was in the middle of her salad. She flirtatiously made him wait until she sipped the noisy bottom bubble of her water through a straw. They both laughed. She enjoyed their comfortable ease and mutual sense of humor. But why rush a leisurely Saturday afternoon? Liz wondered if he had ADHD.

He led her to his car, and she wondered where he'd take her next. She was surprised when he drove into the garage of his townhouse. Again, she joked that now she was entering a strange man's home. Ordinarily, she would never do that on early dates. But he was, after all, the reputed "Great Guy."

His townhouse was overly organized and spacious for one person. Not a paper was out, nor a dish lying around. As though no one lived there, the décor was somber dark browns. Workout equipment was lined up in rows in one room. There were glass enclosed etageres of collectibles, including miniature cars, books, cufflinks, old records in their original and tarnished jackets, and more. Then there was Auntie J's rocking chair, of which Great Guy was very proud, with the fabric worn through. Liz wondered, "What impact did Auntie J have on him?"

Along the walls everywhere were photos of Great Guy from the time he was a baby to the present when he owned his company. The images included his immediate family and long-departed relatives. There were pictures of him with junior high school friends, grandparents, cousins, and distant associations.

This guy lived in the past and kept records! Moreover, everything had a place, and it was obvious there was no place for a woman. His living space screamed, "This is my space, and you're not welcome."

Why did Great Guy invite Liz to see his home? How unorthodox for a first date! Little did he suspect that his man cave foretold his need for control, precision, organization, and protection. No wonder he was unhappy! Structures become strictures, and life's vicissitudes never conform.

Liz had not seen someone in his 60s so precise, anal, and "elderly" in a buff man's body. Because of their high level of rapport, she suspected he was a deep old soul having a depressive, lonely time on Planet Earth.

Still, he was very accommodating. He said, "You ought to come over sometime and watch the stars with me in my garden." Unaware of exactly where she was, she responded, "I don't think I'd know how to find this place again." He graciously offered, "I'll pick you up." That touched Liz.

The pair continued to talk and sing tunes, and he played his guitar. Then, something touching occurred. Earlier, while they had been eating breakfast, she told Great Guy about her sickly neighbor who had skin hunger from being alone for so long. She added, "Since Covid, so do I!" As the largest organ in the body, the skin's touch is ten times stronger than verbal or emotional cues.

Nothing more was said about her skin hunger, but maybe it registered. In one quiet moment, Great Guy looked at her, pulled her close, and caressed her back and arms. She had earlier expressed what she needed, and he recalled it. She swooned, "That feels so good."

Liz didn't remember how and why they pulled apart. She wondered if this man's compelling effect on her was due to her skin hunger, her loneliness, her being overworked, or the fact that the two of them were lush with mutual electricity. He didn't kiss her, nor did he throw her onto one of his beds. He just hugged and massaged her responsive torso. The time it lasted was too short.

Before she knew it, Great Guy led her to his car, and she wondered what their next adventure would be. He had said he was free Saturday afternoon and evening. Did he make plans since he said that? Had he had enough closeness already?

Great Guy was now dropping her off in front of her house. He got out of his side of the car, came around, and opened her car door. She got out, and they again hugged. This time, he gave her a pillowy kiss. No tongue-in-mouth grabby sex kiss. This kiss was nothing she could remember from her past. After unwantedly being mauled by men for years, this kiss was tender. At once, she felt their intoxicating chemistry. He whispered, "Would you like to do this again?" She breathed, "I'd love to."

As soon as she entered her house, she sat on her sofa and stared into space. What just happened? Great Guy warmed her in many ways! And that pillowy kiss punctuated the feeling. Men take merely 15 minutes to decide whether to see a woman a second time. Liz must have passed that threshold since they were together for 2½ hours.

She later texted Great Guy a thank you for their fun afternoon. He replied that it was very "entertaining." He then said he just returned from playing two hours of tennis. Again, Liz wondered if this guy had ADHD. When he asked to see her again, she presumed he meant it. They texted back and forth with some trivial banter, and that was it.

Days went by. There was no contact. Weeks went by. No contact. Months went by. Still no contact. Liz was sad that this man turned out to be shut down. She never heard from him again. Some "Great" Guy!

Liz wondered what happened. The same protective wall that blocks disappointment also blocks happiness. Great Guy's somber brown decor suggested emptiness. He had said he wanted to find an honest and deep relationship. From their first texts, Liz and Great Guy both knew they were on the same page.

To allow love in, a man must be vulnerable enough to be known. Researcher Brene Brown says, "Vulnerability is not winning or losing; it's having the courage to show up and be seen authentically when we have no control over the outcome."

Brown's word "courage" should be emphasized. We're human, we take risks, we screw up. But only when we're authentically open to sharing these experiences can we have deep relationships.

Great Guy didn't even come close to that. When someone

is ashamed of his flaws, he acts unworthy of love, and then he sabotages his relationships. This sabotage usually isn't a conscious or deliberate act but a natural reflex for protection.

People don't express their real emotions because they fear disapproval, hurting others, or adverse consequences like being canceled, punished, or rejected. Since Liz had no idea about Great Guy's history, she couldn't know his fears.

Insecure guys narcissistically concentrate so much on the obstacles that they miss the opportunities to get the love they want. But a man who's "all take" and "no give" would find it impossible to attract a grounded woman who wants an empathic partner.

Gilda-Gram
Empathy is the antidote to shame.

Great Guy asked Liz to see him again, but apparently, he didn't mean it. He was a people pleaser who didn't know how to disconnect gracefully. He could easily lie about being happy on a date because he had plenty of practice putting on a cheery disposition during an unhappy 32-year marriage. Singer and songwriter Jim Morrison wrote, "Most people love you for who you pretend to be. To keep their love, you keep pretending—performing. You get to love your pretense. We're locked in an image, an act."

Remaining in a marriage without the comfort of sharing your honest feelings is self-abuse.

Great Guy was charming, low-key, smooth, and believable,

so he could readily pull off the rouse. But he was stuck. She wondered if he knew it. Men may enjoy superficial games, but women want truth. Liz saw Great Guy as a baby playing love games. She wanted a Real Man.

The Mouths of Innocence
Question: What do most people do on a date?
"On the first date, they tell each other lies,
and that usually gets them interested enough
to go on a second date."
—Martin, Age 10

Great Guy even had his friend Carolyn fooled. For decades, the shellshock of camouflaging his feelings exacerbated his current fear of not feeling good enough for love. Carolyn offered to contact Great Guy to find out what was up with him. Liz said, "Let the hunter hunt. If a man doesn't have enough drive to hunt for what he wants, he doesn't want it badly enough. If a man doesn't want me badly enough, I don't want him."

Great Guy said he wanted love. But as LeAnn Rimes' song "Give" explains, "If you want to get love, then give it." A smart guy advertised on his dating profile, "Tell me what you give, not what you've got."

Before he reached the corner of Kiss and Run, did Great Guy even know that giving was a mandate? Eventually, when a ghost gets out of the Witness Protection Program, he may run out of reasons to run.

Garrison Keillor writes, "Some luck lies in not getting what you thought you wanted, but getting what you have, which once you have it, you may be smart enough to see is what you would have wanted had you known." If only we could be "smart enough" in advance!

CHAPTER 17

Comatose Shutdown

Another way hetero men self-protect is by shutting down their emotions into barren deadness, so they won't feel and thereby hurt. Evolved women walk away from shut down men.

Former New York City mayor Bill de Blasio is still married but separated from his wife while still living with her. Meanwhile, he's on the town as a bachelor. He was spotted with a new girlfriend who is also still married. She claims she is in the process of getting a divorce. When a reporter contacted her husband, physician Owen Stark, in Michigan and asked if Kristy was his ex-wife, he said, "No, that's my wife." He said they weren't in an open marriage, and "she's denied any sort of infidelity in the past. If she has something to tell me, she'll tell me. I haven't seen any legal communication or been made aware of anything like that. You know as much or more than I do at this point."

Photos of his wife and de Blasio canoodling in New York were published, yet this physician father of two sounded comatose to what was happening. No wonder she went looking elsewhere.

In his song, "She Wouldn't Be Gone," the hot masculine cowboy, Blake Shelton, moans regretfully that he was selfish. He took his lady for granted, she warned him to change but he didn't, and she booked. Now, he is desperate to get her back. People want most what they no longer have.

With the woke agenda around him and aggressive females who took the reins, Tim was surprised to date a woman and not receive a call from *her* to ask him out again. Meanwhile, if a date had gone well, the woman's girlfriends would ask, as girlfriends do, "Did you hear from Tim?" Tim knew the expectations but was adamant to pull an obstinate tantrum when he was required to become a vigorous male in pursuit. Some of his dates would not play the woke game of calling him. One woman told him to get potty-trained.

Since the end of COVID, the nation's psychological fallout of being cooped up for years has yielded an epidemic of loneliness. In New York City alone, health surveys found that 57 percent of residents felt lonely sometimes, and 67 percent felt socially isolated. Only a third of those surveyed named someone they could count on for emotional support, and 20 percent reported depression.

PBS News reported, "American men are stuck in what's been dubbed a friendship recession, with 20 percent of single men now saying they don't have any close friends." Saturday Night Live spoofed this dangerous issue with a sketch of a woman escorting her boyfriend to a "man park," similar to a dog park, where he could befriend other guys. The sketch went viral because it struck such a familiar cord regarding men's loneliness.

Loneliness is linked with inflammation and elevated stress hormones that could increase blood pressure. Despite alarming findings, no medical diagnosis or screening for loneliness exists. Not everyone can be so lucky to find a caring Dr. Robert Levine who doused Mary Tyler Moore's loneliness problem.

The condition also affects animals. Known as "the world's saddest elephant," Asian elephant Mali briefly shared her space with another elephant named Shiba. After Shiba died in 1990, Mali lived alone in her pen for 33 years. At Manila Zoo in the Philippines, animal activists Jane Goodall and Paul McCartney pleaded with authorities to transfer Mali to an elephant sanctuary. PETA agreed that she deserved better. Their pleas were ignored. Mali died alone.

Loneliness strikes everyday folks and celebrities alike. Priscilla Presley recalled how she met 24-year-old Elvis when she was just 14. Not being sexual at her young age, she said her role was to listen to The King pour out his heart as a "very, very lonely" young man in 1959.

I understand Elvis' loneliness. I was a star on stage while the audience held onto my every word. But then when the adoring audience was gone, the stage was quiet, and I suddenly felt empty. I consulted my Broadway actress friend. She explained that my empty feelings were typical of all performers after the circus leaves town. Performers experience the adrenalin rush, but then feel the depletion when it ends. I discovered it the hard way.

A 2022 Psychology Today article, "What's Behind the Rise of Lonely, Single Men?" exposed the reality that dating opportunities for heterosexual men are diminishing as relationship standards rise. While 64 percent of dating apps are comprised of men, women are more selective. They no longer need a man to raise a child or support them financially. The article pointed out that younger and middle-aged men are the loneliest they have been in years, and it predicted the situation would get worse. Being in a relationship isn't a solution for happiness—and being with the wrong mate could have the opposite effect. But statistics show that men's physical and emotional health improve when they're paired with a loving partner.

However, women with good educations and higher salaries have become more selective in demanding that partners be emotionally available and able to communicate openly. Boys are usually not taught the basics for sustaining relationships. Mature women today have little patience for shut-down, cloistered men.

Sun Tzu
"If victory is long in coming,
weapons will grow dull, and ardor will be dampened."

The Psychology Today article advised men to seek therapy and get to know, accept, and share who they are. That won't happen while men are finding ways to hide and mute their pain. For example, why get therapy when men feel their sexual needs are being satisfied through porn? Sadly, young men often believe that sex is the only reason for sustaining a relationship!

In 2016, Pew Research Center found that for the first time in the modern era, living with parents eclipsed living with an intimate partner for millennial 18- to 34-year-olds. This situation has increased since the pandemic. I've met older men, too, who live not with a mate but with a parent, with the excuse that they are their parents' caregiver. Or is it the other way around?

Richard Reeves is the author of "Of Boys and Men" and the director of the Men and Boys Project at the Brookings Institution, where he is a Senior Fellow. He notes that men account for almost three of four "deaths of despair" through alcohol-related illness, suicide, or drug overdose. It's healthful and helpful that some celebrity men are broadcasting their depression so other men might realize they, too, need help. However, as more women dominate the labor force, the shrinking numbers of men on the job push men to question why they exist.

Unbeknownst to most, even Santa's reindeer are female; that's the gender of the deer population that keeps its antlers during the winter. Deer with the largest antlers are socially dominant and more physically fit—and in this case, they're girls!

In the human world, the female-to-male imbalance is not getting better. Reeves notes that "the 2020 decline in college enrollment was seven times greater for males than for females in the United States." In academia, I see a dramatic increase in female college and graduate students, which was not the case years ago. Today, a primary goal in all universities is student retention, which keeps an institution solvent. I was offered a high-salaried position as Dean of Student Retention, which I declined because I don't want to be counting when I can be communicating.

Reeves and I had similar motives for writing our books. Reeves said that we've finally opened opportunities for girls and women—but that doesn't mean we should forget boys and men. Similarly, I say that we've finally opened opportunities for LGBTQ+s—but that doesn't mean we should forget hetero boys and men.

Why does it have to be one group to the exclusion of the other? The corpus callosum is the band that joins the right and left hemispheres of the brain. Its thickness in men can disrupt walking and talking simultaneously because it's challenging to go from left to right quickly. Its thinness in women encourages burnout from multitasking a job, a house, and parenting. Neither gender benefits from being in the shadows.

In a CNN interview, Reeves said Democrats are reluctant to

deemphasize women and LGBTQ+s for fear they'll offend those who have already been offended for centuries. But Washington Post writer Christine Embe warns that masculinity defined solely to denigrate women propels male defensiveness and victimization.

Disagreement is where the plight of the hetero man in trouble shows itself. New lovers T.J. Holmes and Amy Robach discussed their arguing styles on their podcast. He admitted he "checks out" with an "I'm done," and that's the end. He said, "I don't scream, I don't yell, I don't do anything. I don't name-call, I don't get aggressive, nothing. I don't need you to say, 'I'm sorry.' I don't need you to help me. I have to work through it, and I'm trying to get better at doing it quicker." T.J. admitted he would have 18 drinks in one day before he recognized he needed to do something about his "relationship with alcohol." Not unlike many men, he becomes a comatose shut-down.

Robach lamented, "It's two days, at least," until he comes around. "I would rather have him yell at me than freeze me out for two days. I don't know what to say or do or what he thinks." Instead of leveling with him about his freeze-out, she began imbibing 30 drinks a week, which is not healthy for someone who overcame cancer.

Why do men shut down during crises? It's self-protection, and for some, it may be because the conflict reminds them of their critical mother from days gone by. Conflict demands discussion—hopefully, before two days have passed. But the length of the silence depends on each person's Propinquity Quotient, another discussion couples omit.

Most men haven't learned or practiced fair fighting techniques that employ "When you..., I felt..." constructions. So, they feel victimized and look for cover to protect themselves from Mama's wrath. Sadly, it is typical to repeat the same fight throughout an entire relationship.

The fear of Mama's wrath is especially noteworthy for boys and men. Embe's findings, similar to those of others researched here, say that since 1960, the percentage of fatherless boys rose from 17 percent to 32 percent. Where is a male to go if Mama (or a Mama figure) withdraws love for any reason? That's a very frightening thought that many men pack with them into adulthood. If his father left, what's to say his mother would not do the same?

To prevent mom's defection, some men overly attach to a maternal standard no other woman can meet. On one dating site, the very first photo a 70-year-old man advertised showed him beside his elderly mother. Were he and Mom a package deal?

There may be another side of the coin for a grown man to live with his mother. A reporter asked 38-year-old Portuguese footballer Cristiano Ronaldo, "Why does your mother still live with you? Why not build her a house?"

He replied, "My mother raised me by sacrificing her life for me. She slept hungry so I could eat at night. We had no money at all. She worked seven days a week and evenings as a cleaner to buy my first football equipment so that I could become a player. My complete success is dedicated to her. And as long as I live, she will always be by my side and have everything I can give her. She is my refuge and my greatest gift."

Ronaldo's father died at 52 of an alcohol-related illness. Although he hasn't married, he has five children, has custody of one, and continues to have female relationships. Grandma is a constant, and everyone accepts the setup. In large spaces, this is not impossible.

Besides those men living with their mothers, other men grow up fearing that some woman will leave them. Preventatively, they either avoid deep relationships altogether or take the first step to antagonize those they have to avoid getting dumped.

Many of the men Embe interviewed had troubled relationships with their dads or no father figure at all. Farrell notes that seven out of eight boys involved in school shootings are dad deprived. He says, "Women have women centers and men also have men's centers. They're called prisons, or centers for dad-deprived boys."

Young men would benefit from reading Robert Bly's classic, "Iron John: A Book about Men" that discusses remote fatherhood. Richard Reeves says there's a good chance these boys won't meet a male figure until middle school. Bly, Embe, and Reeves agree that virtuous male role models help boys thrive. I say they help males *survive*.

Do men become comatose shutdowns so as not to offend the

women with whom they're arguing? Where does men's silence leave the world? A solution to discord only emerges through open and honest dialogue, but not too long after a wound.

Reeves said that in every advanced economy in the world today, there are more women than men with a college degree, at the ratio of 60:40. How will this eventually play out in the relationship sector, knowing that women have become more selective, while men are isolating and finding dangerous alternative escapes from intimacy? In time, with disparate educations, will a female physician feel intellectually compatible with and want to marry a lineman with a high school diploma? Reeves says we don't know that yet. I think we do.

As the independence and selectivity of women continue, there will be fewer eligible men in the coral, and women, too, will end up similarly single and lonely. An educated but lonely attorney in his 70s recently revealed that he could partner with a less-educated hairdresser, seamstress, or cashier. Thus, there may be two standards for choosing mates: one for evolved women and one for lonely men.

Loneliness findings are not isolated to the United States. In 2021, Japan appointed a minister of loneliness to overcome its burgeoning suicide rate. Still, nothing is formally being done. The great irony is that while people are lonely, many also fear getting close!

A man online posted this: "Walking through my son's schoolyard, I noticed a bench painted bright red. I asked my son, 'Is that the only place to sit around here?'

He said, 'No, that's the buddy bench. When someone feels lonely, or they have nobody to play with, they sit there, and kids ask them to play.'

I asked if he ever used it.

He said, 'Yeah. When I was new, I sat there, and someone came and asked me to play. I felt happy. And now, when I see kids on it, I ask them to play with me. We all do.'"

Children employ sensitive outreaches that grownups somehow miss. Are men brave enough to discard their closeted hurts and leap toward openness and interaction? Due to identity fears, too many heterosexual men are reluctant to speak up. The longer men feel declining self-worth, the lonelier they become and the more they self-protect and eventually self-destruct.

<u>Gilda-Gram</u>
**We won't know how to help anyone
until we agree that we all need help.**

Help begins with helping ourselves first. At 46, former playboy John Mayer announced that he was retired from bachelorhood and bed-mating, and was ready to get married. He said he believes "that level of being relied on is the hottest thing in the world." Although it sounds naive, he said, he'd like to hear his wife say, "Call John. Call my husband. You're a full grown-up when this is your romantic fantasy." He said he quit drinking six years ago, and now he wants a wife and family life. Instead of looking for a quickie, he sleeps with a row of pillows on the other side of the bed.

When Mayer does finally tie the knot, his former girlfriends from Taylor Swift to Katy Perry may be singing Jana Kramer's song, "I Got the Boy, She Got the Man." John Mayer proves there's always a chance for the comatose to awaken.

CHAPTER 18

Long Distance Sprinter

The longer the trek, the greater the yearning. The greater the yearning, the more erotic the fantasy.

The more erotic the fantasy . . . Stop there! Once the long-distance fantasy becomes a reality, you're left with big travel bills, airline delays, time changes, weather snags, and aborted communications. Long distance relationships can't work long term unless one person intends to move, and the pair starts anew in a residence that is jointly theirs. People settled in successful careers rarely opt to topple their hard-earned achievements for a relocation.

After the termination of a failed long distance relationship, Dee was vacationing in a boutique hotel in Santa Monica habituated by beautiful, tanned Europeans. As she waited by the elevator bank to go to her room, out of the corner of her eye, she saw a man walking her way. Waiting for the elevator to arrive at the lobby where she would get in, Full Frontal was taking long strides toward her.

There's staring—and then there's ocular intrusion. Before Dee could blink, this man was in her personal space. He introduced himself and showered the woman with endless compliments. This tall, dapper man had a distinguished British accent. He invited Dee for coffee. She declined, saying there was no point because they lived oceans away. He tried to convince her otherwise and asked for her phone number. She smiled, apologized, and knew she'd never repeat a long distance romance. She walked into the elevator and pressed a different floor than her own to guarantee her safety.

Unless it's because of a work situation, long distance relationships are unconsciously set up because one or both people in a couple have low Propinquity Scores. With distance, they can play at dating and loving from afar while drinking in the excitement of new beginnings. They know that unless one of the pair is willing to relocate—and the other wants that to happen—the relationship can only be fantasy. Long distance is hot, but it's also inconvenient.

One couple who met the challenges of long distance sprinting were two people I set up on a blind date. Sarah, a mathematics genius, was getting her doctorate with me at New York University. Sol, a bookish brainiac with a penchant for science, knew my husband at the time.

Because Sarah was writing her doctoral dissertation, she was unwilling to meet Sol or any other man until she completed Chapter 5. Sol joked that his whole love life was being put on ice for Chapter 5. When the pair finally did meet, sparks flew, as I knew they would. He was the director of a large hospital laboratory, and Sarah was teaching at a university while completing her Ph.D. dissertation. They were engaged that year and married six months later.

After two years of wedded bliss, Sol decided to attend medical school. But he was already 35, and American medical schools would not accept him. So, he applied to and was accepted at a med school in Guadalajara, Mexico.

For four grueling years, the couple commuted from Mexico to New York. Sol had to learn medical terminology in Spanish and English and go into the dangerous mountains to treat indigent Mexicans in need of medical care. One year, Sarah moved to Mexico to be with her husband. But money was tight, and she had to return to the States where she could make somewhat of a living to support them as they got further into debt.

Somehow, the couple managed the distance, and Sol returned to the U.S., took his medical boards, and began a practice as an anesthesiologist. Along came two children, and the rest is history. How many couples can survive such hardships? This couple had no choice but to be apart, but they knew that eventually, the time away from each other would end, and they would be together again.

Usually, when a long distance couple begins playing, they aren't in a deeply committed relationship. Passion is driving their train, and the long distance adds to the exhilaration, like the endorphins built up from sneaking around when cheating.

The heat might not be so intense if two people were in the same neighborhood without the intrigue. By the time my friends went long distance, they were already married, they mutually committed to putting Sol through med school, and they worked as a team to manifest their goals.

Tonya and Marty met while she lived in Los Angeles, and he was in Phoenix. Their commute was only an hour by air or a six-hour drive. For two years, they met for trips to Europe, going skiing, boating, and sightseeing. Tonya wanted Marty to move to California while she knew he had a great job as president of a large company in Phoenix. Marty wanted Tonya to move to Phoenix, while he knew she had a one-of-a-kind position that was her dream of a lifetime. Neither was willing to leave their coveted jobs. When Marty described their breakup, he seemed angry. Why? They both knew the end was inevitable. In truth, long distance sprinters are more commitment-phobic than they admit!

Sure, we saw the story of Prince Harry leave the Royals for Meghan Markle. And Edward VIII, King of the United Kingdom of Great Britain and Northern Ireland and Emperor of India, abdicated his throne in 1936 for the American woman he loved, Wallis Warfield Simpson, who was still married to her second husband. Then there are the mushy Hallmark movies where one prince or another breaks protocol to claim the hand of some American country bumpkin.

The unconscious drive for the insecure is "if he leaves his life for me, that's proof I'm great." But love is not about proving one's greatness. We're supposed to enter a relationship with that already as a given. Love is about having a soul connection and intertwining lives. Yet, grown women still sing Disney's fantasy tune, hoping, "Someday, my prince will come."

Legendary Disney filmmaker John Musker has called out the Mouse House for having gone too woke. He said the formula should consist of story over political agenda, and Disney has inverted its priorities. Kids—and adults—still trust these films to be their destiny.

At the last minute, a New York paparazzi friend grabbed me to accompany her to parties she was covering for the night. I was not dressed for a formal occasion, wearing a brown crushed velvet floor length dress I had bought in an upscale consignment shop on a whim. It was too big on top and kept falling off my shoulders. I was also carrying an unsightly Bag Lady tote. It was not exactly socialite couture. But this invitation necessitated me to come as I was dressed.

We landed at the Waldorf Astoria at The Princess Grace Awards. A man in a tux with whom I did business spotted me when I exited the elevator. He asked whether I wanted to meet Prince Albert since this man had just returned from business meetings in Monaco, and he knew the prince well. I told him, "No, thank you. Royalty is not my thing."

But before I knew it, the man had my arm looped in his, and he delivered me to the prince as "The Love Doc," my title when I hosted the MTV Show by that name. The prince was holding court among throngs of admirers. He immediately turned to me and smiled broadly, saying, "I need to get some pointers from you." I laughed, "I don't think you need pointers from me. I haven't followed your life, but the few headlines I've seen suggest you're doing just fine in that department." I poked fun at his thinking he needed a love doc for any purpose.

I knew some of the surrounding female swooners vying to become Cinderella. There was a circle of sparkling, beautiful New Yorkers, socialites, and paparazzi, and everyone (except me) was perfectly bedecked. But they watched Prince Albert ask *me* for my phone number! I refused repeatedly. The more I refused, the more he lobbied for my digits. The paparazzi moved closer to hear our banter. So, to tease them more, the prince playfully whispered in my ear. We had a fun repartee, and the rubbernecking media were desperate with curiosity.

Some notables later asked how I charmed the prince. Ha! In my too-big dress and Bag Lady tote, I told the onlookers I didn't know what to say, so I told him I had written a book about him: "Don't Bet on the Prince!" I quickly yanked a postcard of the book cover from that unsightly tote. The prince held it between us as he put his arm around me. The paparazzi shot a photo of it and the photo made its rounds through Europe. Since my book was published in multiple languages, that unintentional shot did wonders for my worldwide book sales. I had lost myself in spur-of-the-moment, devil-may-care amusement to hide my ill-prepared feelings and my inadequate costume.

After our meeting, the prince and I had great interchanges,

including a laugh-filled four-hour phone conversation from his location in Paris to mine in New York. He has a great sense of humor, is brilliantly informed and worldly, and he actually read "Don't Bet on the Prince!" before taking me to dinner when he returned to the States. I knew he had read the book because he commented on how accurate my description of Princess Di had been and wondered how I knew. We discussed my third eye insight, and he wanted to bring me to Monaco to work with his Royal family.

Then, his father, Prince Rainier, the late Princess Grace Kelly's husband, suddenly passed. Albert had a throne to take over, so our future became history. However, even with our intriguing interactions, the distance would have precluded a forever after—unless I chose to convert my 1300 square foot "palace" into his real one. Despite all the seemingly magical frills, I knew I could never take on a *role* that would overshadow a *relationship*, despite how connected we felt.

Long distance sets up unrealistic futures—and hurts. Fantasies are vital for a child's healthy development, but a rational adult must accept the excruciating nature of this setup. To prevent hurt feelings from setting in, couples must honestly share what they want. But more importantly, they must come clean about what they are prepared to sacrifice.

PART IV
SOLUTIONS FOR EMOTIONAL DETOX

CHAPTER 19

Toxic Men in Trouble

These days, red-blooded men almost expect to be maligned for being men. Many are fed up with their less-than-flattering stereotypes, being painted into categories, discriminated against, and having injustices lodged against them for acts they never committed. They see woke men being ridiculed, but they are also turned off by the large number of abhorrent toxic males in the news. Here are some of the big names finally being made to pay for their toxicity:

- Hollywood producer Harvey Weinstein was sent to prison for 23 years for rape and sexual abuse.

- A graduate of the Yale School of Drama, accomplished actor Jonathan Majors was accused by ex-girlfriend Grace Jabbari of smashing household objects against the wall of their bedroom in fits of rage. After showing jurors a dent he left in the wall, she said, "His face just kind of changes when he gets into that place."

Majors was convicted of assault and harassment charges against his former girlfriend. Then this tough supervillain was dumped by Marvel Studios owned by Disney, and he was dropped by his publicists, his management company, and his talent agency. He also faced up to a year in jail. This actor was a rising star, and Disney had great plans for him for the next several years. A source said, "You can get away with a lot of things in Hollywood. But hitting your girlfriend isn't one of them."

• Federal investigators found that former New York Governor Mario Cuomo sexually harassed at least 13 women he employed and retaliated against ex-staff members. This created a hostile work environment in the governor s office. Although he denied the charges, it was reported that he "repeatedly subjected female employees to unwelcome, non-consensual sexual contact, ogling, unwelcome sexual comments, gender-based nicknames, comments on their physical appearances, and/or preferential treatment based on their physical appearances." A few of Cuomo's accusers are also pursuing their own legal action against him.

• After decades of rumors about his violent behavior, 54-year-old Puff Daddy or P. Diddy was sued by his former girlfriend, 37-year-old R & B singer Cassie (Cassandra Ventura), for repeatedly raping her, physically abusing her, and forcing her to have sex with male prostitutes while he watched and masturbated. The two had been a couple from 2007 to 2018. She described his "uncontrollable rage" and his beatings.

Just 24 hours after the suit had been filed it was settled. The hashtag #SurvivingDiddy began trending on X with the prediction that more women would come forward. Then after eight years of vehemently denying the accusations, a 2016 video surfaced of him brutally beating and dragging Cassie. The video was so vivid, Combs issued a hollow apology on Instagram: "It's so difficult to reflect on the darkest times in your life, but sometimes you got to do that. I was f—ed up. I hit rock bottom — but I make no excuses. My behavior on that video is inexcusable. I take full responsibility for my actions. I'm disgusted." I told the National Enquirer the only thing the rapper was sorry for was being caught on tape.

Combs used his wealth and influence to control Ventura, whom he met when she was 19 and he was 37. She was signed with Combs' label, so they were also in business together through 2019. Women often remain with brutes because they don't believe they can make it on their own. Is it worth the fear, the cuts, the bruises?

With enough digging, Ventura would have learned that Combs had a history of violence with women, even beating his college girlfriend with a belt while others watched aghast. His domestic abuse continued for years without consequence— until everyone saw it on tape. Now he may rot in jail for racketeering and sex trafficking!

- On the TV show, "So You Think You Can Dance," Paula Abdul sued film director Nigel Lythgoe, alleging he sexually assaulted her in a hotel elevator while they were traveling for "American Idol" during the show's early beginnings. Court documents say Lythgoe shoved Abdul against a wall, grabbed her genitals and breasts and shoved his tongue down her mouth. I ended when the elevator door opened, and Abdul escaped to her hotel room and called her representative in tears.

On another occasion, Abdul attended a dinner she believed was for professional purposes at Lythgoe's home. She alleged that he jumped on her, proposing they would make a good "power couple." She escaped as soon as she threw him off her.

Lythgoe denied the accusations and said that for two decades the pair worked as dear platonic friends, and he is shocked and saddened by the accusations.

Then two other "Jane Does" filed suits against Lythgoe with similar accusations that occurred during another competition show, "All American Girl," which aired in 2003. They allege Lythgoe "walked around the set and dressing rooms and openly swatted and groped" their buttocks. They said he also "made sexual advances" on them at his home.

Lythgoe stepped down as a judge on "So You Think You Can Dance" right after the Abdul lawsuit so he could "clear his name and restore his reputation."

- Vince McMahon was a powerful behemoth of a man accused of sexual assault and trafficking. He denied the allegations, but he left his position as executive chairman of WWE-parent TKO Group Holdings amid a sexual abuse and trafficking scandal that rocked the world of wrestling.

As the co-founder of the modern WWE, McMahon was sued by ex-staffer Janel Grant alleging that he defecated on her during a threesome, trafficked her to other WWE executives, and sexually abused her with sex toys that caused her injuries. WWE president and TKO board member Nick Khan said, "McMahon will no longer have a role with TKO Group Holdings or WWE."

McMahon allegedly promised naïve Grant a job with the company after her parents died. The job entailed having a sexual relationship with him, which continued into January 2022.

He then shared nude photos of her to other employees and directed her to have sex with other executives and a wrestling star. The lawsuit also alleges that McMahon texted Grant in 2020: "I'm the only one who owns U and controls who I want to f—."

* * *

Toxic violations of women are such common occurrences that when a man *doesn't* annoy an attractive woman, he actually gets praised. A woman was admiring her graduation outfit in a store mirror. A man outside the store smoked a cigarette while his eyes lingered on the woman's body. The response to the clip amassed over 27 million views. People praised the ocular intruder for being respectful of the woman's boundaries for not approaching her.

Years ago, when it felt safe to talk to strangers on a big city street, I was looking in a shop window on New York's elegant Madison Avenue. While lost in admiring the dreamy goods, a man approached me from behind and chided, "See anything you like?" Without missing a beat, and never turning around to see who I was answering, I smiled and joked, "You buying?"

I turned around, he was a well-dressed lawyer, we walked, we talked, we went for coffee, and we had some dates. That was then. These days, if a strange man tried to engage me on a city street, I would run for safety! What was once fun repartee between genders has morphed into danger and distrust.

In contrast to being a brute, being woke is the other end of the spectrum. Acknowledging the need for an alternative path to what exists, 30-year-old New Yorker, Niko Emanuilidis, with no psychology training, is teaching men how to have "daddy" energy when looking for love. He defines that quality as a confident, caring alpha without the angry edge. Demonstrating respect for women, these "daddies make ladies feel safe and at ease." He names Travis Kelce as a "daddy."

Woke men often wait for the female to take the lead. Travis is of the woke generation, yet he aggressively pursued Taylor Swift through many different channels until he finally made contact. He admits he followed a strategy. He put in the effort to get to know and understand her. He wasn't intimidated by her star power. He inconvenienced himself to attend her shows around the world, wherever she was performing. At one show, he dismissed her bodyguard saying, "It's okay. I can take it from here." He's what Emanuilidis calls a "daddy" because he's not afraid to show his emotions for his lady and he doesn't think he's less of a man for making her feel special. That's where all men should be. It's not woke and it's not toxic. Travis's behavior is honest, strategic, assertive, and vulnerable. And that's exactly what most women want in a mate.

After boasting 135,000 followers on TikTok, Emanuilidis opened his Daddy Academy. He teaches women how to recognize mistreatment and men how to be attractively vulnerable. As you've consistently read here, women enjoy strong but vulnerable men who are balanced between work and personal passions. If this street smart dating guru wants to call it "daddy energy" so be it, as long as the end result is men who exude pride in who they are.

Actor Bradley Cooper had to exit a press conference for his new Movie "Maestro" after getting an urgent call from his six-year-old daughter's school's nurse. He shares joint custody of Lea with his ex-girlfriend, model Irina Shayk, with whom he was together for four years. Both Shayk and Cooper have moved on to other mates. But Shayk gushed on Instagram, "So proud of Daddy and Lea." True daddy energy with true female respect.

While the breakups and new couplings of celebrities continue, the "daddy energy" of older guys is admirable.

Seventy-three year old Jay Leno filed for a conservatorship for his wife of 40 years, 77-year-old Mavis who was diagnosed with Alzheimer's. The love this couple has always expressed has been exemplary, but now especially, Leno's devotion reflects "daddy energy" at its best.

CHAPTER 20

Why Do Good Men Stay Silent?

"Hidden in Plain Sight: How Men's Fears of Women Shape their Intimate Relationships" by Avrum Weiss calls out men reluctant to confront abuse, especially if it is from a woman. The book was excerpted in Psychology Today. It said, first, men feel ashamed to admit that they need anything from anyone. Second, there's fear that conflict, criticism, or disapproval will lead to men's abandonment.

There's a third reason for good men's silence not mentioned in the article: men's unwitting suspicion that whoever angers them conquers them. They know the hold their emotions have on them, and they are terrified of being conquered and swallowed up, especially by a woman. So, men are willing to contort themselves to any extent to avoid Mama's wrath reminiscent of their critical mother.

Fear and shame rule—often irrationally. The male praying

mantis cannot copulate while its head is attached to its body, so the female initiates sex by ripping the male's head off. But those are praying mantises, not Real Men! Female mosquitoes bite and drink blood, while wussy male mosquitoes do not bite, but feed on the nectar of flowers. But those are mosquitoes, not Real Men! Female black widow spiders are more dangerous than their male counterparts. They have more prominent venomous glands, longer fangs and a body size that can become up to 20-times larger than the males. But those are spiders, not Real Men! Male bees die after mating. But those are male bees, not Real Men!

Will Smith rationalized Jada's put-downs by telling the New York Times, "When you've been with someone for more than half your life, emotional blindness sets in." Is that why he told the media that Jada is his best friend, and he will remain with her for the rest of his life? He said her revelations made him realize how "resilient, clever, and compassionate" she is. How does a "resilient, clever, and compassionate" woman keep maligning the man she claims to "love deeply"? After being "emotionally blinded," why wasn't his emotional sight restored after he digested the ridicule he suffered as Hollywood's cuckhold?

Over time, people learn to tolerate, trivialize, and hold their numbing pain inside unless they're guided by a therapist. Without support, men in pain are afraid and probably too numb to get close enough to themselves to reveal their deepest angst. Anger is a natural expression about something that is not right. But it's how we manage and deliver our anger that counts. It must be addressed and confronted without explosion so that its message can be interpreted and acted on. This is a learned skill.

Fear and love cannot live under the same roof. Victims don't think they deserve rights, so they develop a high tolerance for hurtful behavior from someone who purports to care. When they realize they've been deceived, their depression becomes even deeper, and they choose to silence themselves more.

CHAPTER 21

Check Your Emotional History

Carolyn Myss, author of "Why People Don't Heal" notes that people speak "woundology" where their painful childhoods become their language of intimacy. They interact by complaining and whining about their issues, and they usually attract like-minded partners and friends. These associations prevent them from breaking the mold. Surrounded by sameness, they don't see their problem until it becomes a crisis.

Long-suffering victims won't heal until the language of woundology is disabled and replaced with one of self-care and love for others. When it's presented to him, will a man recognize a sincere love offer or run from it?

Take inventory of your early interactions by responding to the following questions.

Your Dad

- What did you like best about your dad?
- What did you like least about your dad?
- What have you not communicated to your dad that you want to let him know?
- What did your dad not tell you that you needed to hear?

Other Men

- What do you admire in men today?
- What do you dislike in men today?

Your Mom

- What did you like best about your mom?
- What did you like least about your mom?
- What have you not communicated to your mom that you want to let her know?
- What did your mom not tell you that you needed to hear?

Other Women

- What do you like best about women today?
- What do you like least about women today?

Your Responses

1. What did you discover about yourself from your responses to this inventory?
2. What feelings burble inside that you'd like to get out now?
3. Name three strong words that describe you. Why did you choose each?
4. Match each strong word with an emotion.
5. What did you discover?
6. What would you like your next step in life to be?
7. Identify with one of these three types of personalities:

    A. Those who make life happen.

    B. Those to whom life happens.

    C. Those who sleepwalk into "What happened?"

The first type of person (A) uses action to create destiny with grounded mental health.

The second type of person (B) is the victim, "Woe is me. I'm always unlucky!!"

The third type of person (C) suffers from a variant of DID, Dissociative Identity Disorder, where another identity will provide *a ready escape from negative experiences.* It's the toxic male who obliviously slaps another when his anger runs amok, or the furry who escapes humanity into an animal form, or the people pleaser who grabs love from whomever he can please, or any number of different personas.

Of these three types, (A) is the only authentic persona that will ascend to a danger-free zone of proud achievement.

<u>Gilda-Gram</u>
A crisis can be a turning point
or a breaking point.

We are not on this earth to remain do-nothing intransigents. Letting go is not giving up; it's *growing up* and *going up*.

With no work and a foul reputation in his industry, Will Smith knew he had to grow up after slapgate. Fortunately, he had the mental wherewithal and creativity to launch another plan to remain in the spotlight and regain manly respect. He announced he would return to his roots in the world of rap. How would he handle the potty-mouth rap lyrics he vowed to his grandmother he would never use again? His new venture was a podcast of rap from the 80s that had tamer lyrics than those heard today. It's a first and healthy step away from the bravado of a family façade that never had his back. I hope this is a happily-ever-after story for this dazzling talent.

CHAPTER 22

Simple Steps to Reconstruct a Spine

Men who feel shame and humiliation need to first heal their relationship with *themselves*. That is the same and only self that shows up for all interactions. Ask these questions:

1. **What was done to me?**
   Answer: "I allowed my voice to be silenced."

2. **What did I do about it?**
   Answer: "Nothing."

3. **What did I fail to do?**
   Answer: "I failed to defend my truth by correcting the impression that I am compliant.

The answers to these questions open thoughts for the deep work that must follow.

Gilda-Gram
**We only keep behaviors
that continue to serve us.**

Are your behaviors serving you? Who owns your life? There is always a hidden payoff for continuing to suffer: it's the familiar and secure place where a victim knows what to expect. That's how suffering makes a world predictable, comfortable, and controlled.

Through wisdom or woe, men can choose to get better or get bitter. A victim rarely perceives his own power. Changing your routine is uncomfortable at first. Fold your hands. Which finger is on top? Change it. Note how uncomfortable that change feels!

People lie to serve a purpose. Probe the payoff derived from maintaining a façade. This is your doorway to pain management.

1. **Question**: "Pain, what is the payoff I derived from keeping you around?"

    Answer: "I believe I deserve this pain because..." (Clue: When were you *first* rewarded for swallowing your feelings rather than exposing them?)

2. **Question**: Where did you usually bury your feelings? In childhood? In marriage? In school? In parenting? At work? How did each burial work for you?

    Answer: "I would be happier now if..."

Gilda-Gram
**We are trapped by WHO we are
not WITH WHOM we stay.**

The 2004 movie "What the Bleep Do We Know?" teaches that most people write an intention—only to erase it quickly. For that reason, deeper questions like these should follow:

3. **Question**: "Pain, what information can you give me?"

    Answer: "Living a lie has destroyed my sense of self. I want my family and my kids to feel proud of me."

4. **Question**: "Pain, how must I prepare to let you go?"

    Answer: "Rather than being pissed off about my pain, I will expose my truth. Before I have a bond with another person, I must first own a healthy, worthy self that upholds my freedom."

5. **Question**: "Pain, how can I eliminate my bad memories?"

    Answer: "I will list the negative labels someone has called me: 'She says I am . . .' I will then list the positive labels I can use to describe myself: 'I know I am . . .' Study the contrast between the two lists.

6. **Question**: "Pain, how can I keep you at bay?"

   Answer: "I will look beyond the comfort of my irrational behavior. I will ask myself, 'Is this part of a loving and respectful relationship?' 'Does anyone have the right to treat me this way?' I will not be angry with myself. I will stop negative thoughts that induce negative emotions and replace them with positive thoughts that nurture me."

7. **Question**: "Pain, how can I stop my tormentor from repeating her abuse?"

   Answer: It's my behavior, not my words, that tells people what they can and can't get away with. It's okay to have fears of being abandoned or engulfed, but I won't let them dominate or direct me."

Writer W. Somerset Maugham advised, "It's a very funny thing about life; if you refuse to accept anything but the best, you very often get it."

8. **Question**: "Pain, what must I do to finally let you go?"

   Answer: "I must reveal my shame story and share my truth."

Gilda-Gram
Healing occurs when we share our story.

On X, writer and trauma survivor Nate Postlethwait posted, "People don't talk about how painful it is to come alive. By revealing your story, you are forced to start naming what shut off your heart." People pleasers who don't share their truth are emotionally dysfunctional. To keep everyone happy, they don't remember which lie they told to which person. It becomes confusing to the pleaser and it's a communications rip-off to all involved.

In contrast, transparency lets anger and grief breathe freely without shame.

Stories punctuate the Bible, the oldest book of all time. People remember stories because they tap emotions. Walt Disney's approach was to switch positions with the audience and see a story from its point of view. Great salespeople employ this technique. We can't change our true story, but after we share it, we can re-write our future with a happier destiny.

No sane person wants to hurt someone deliberately. But people hurt others because they themselves are hurting. Couples should try role reversal. A woman might get into the shoes of her man to feel the full spectrum of the damage she is doing. The man should don the shoes of his woman to understand why she is so angry and demeaning. Role reversals can powerfully trump the humiliating accusations and put-downs anyone has doled out. Hugh Prather's "Notes to Myself" asks, "If we can make our loved ones unhappy, why don't we work to make them happy?"

Love cannot survive as a Cheerio, with a physically airbrushed exterior but an emotionally hollow center. If we don't talk it out, we'll inevitably act it out. And we'll be sorry.

Lord, grant me the serenity to accept the things I cannot change, the courage to change the things I cannot accept, and the wisdom to protect the hearts of those I crushed because they pissed me off!

Sadly, most people merge lives without having a solid sense of who they are. It takes women seven attempts to leave an abusive relationship. One in six or seven men are abused compared to one in four women. Unlike women, 49 percent of men fail to tell anyone, and 11 percent contemplate suicide. The reaction to domestic violence is devastating to men already questioning their masculinity. Men tend to hide and suffer their shame alone. But because we attract who we are, not who we want, every relationship must begin with a strong Capital "I."

In contrast,

Gilda-Gram
"i love you" with a lower-case "i"
attracts lower-case losers.

We first make our habits, then our habits make us. Difficulties that are mastered are opportunities that are won. It takes time, but to create a healthy relationship from one that's been tattered, two people must lay out their truths. The Sedona Method asks, "Could I let it go?" "Would I?" "When?" Personally, I deliberately surround myself with people who are happily coupled so I breathe in respectful love around me that I can model.

Most people have old mindsets and habits set up over decades that need to be dismantled. That could take time. Elisabeth Kübler-Ross names five phases to process a goodbye before new life can emerge:

1. Denial
2. Anger
3. Bargaining
4. Depression
5. Acceptance

With all our historical insecurities, before we say, "I Do" we must say, "I Count." Being unmarried can shorten a man's life by 10 years. But being married to someone who humiliates him will shorten his lifespan by more.

People can't heal what they don't feel. There is never shame in feeling your worth. If a man needs "crutches" with people who care about him, that's when he can safely ask for directions!

Sun Tzu
"If you know the enemy and know yourself,
you need not fear the result of a hundred battles."

Some shame is legitimate healthy shame, which is the normal human emotion that lets you know you can make a mistake and still feel okay. Its adage is, "I made a mistake. So what?" But unhealthy shame hides honest vulnerability through coverups, overeating, drugs, porn, people pleasing and other mechanisms in a game of make-believe. That kind of shame screams, "I AM a mistake." And that message is projected to all you meet.

<u>Gilda-Gram</u>
To heal shame,
emerge from hiding!

Sisters and brothers, raise up your hands, for we have seen the light!

In an episode on the Showtime series "Homeland," Brody's broken wife said, "For the longest time, all I wanted was for you to tell me the truth. I wanted to know it all. Carrie knows, right? She knows everything about you. She accepts it. You must love her a lot."

Yes, Brody had opened his secrets to Carrie, but not to his wife.

The greatest aphrodisiac is to know and be known by a partner. It's the glue that keeps a relationship bonded and free from extraneous entities. Brody's wife did not experience that with her husband—but the woman with whom he worked, Carrie, did. The wife's pain was palpable.

In the last episode of Season 2 of "Homeland," viewers see how truth is love:

Carrie to Brody: "We have no secrets now."

Brody: "Where's your mom now?"

Carrie: "The day I left for college, she said she was going to CVS. She never came back."

Brody: "And your mom now? Has she reached out to you since?"

Carrie: "That part does hurt."

Brody: "Thanks for telling me."

Carrie: "You're the first one."

He tenderly takes her face in his hands.

Later, Carrie says, "I can't see into your f—king soul, Brody."

Brody replies, "Yes you can."

The only reason Carrie was able to know Brody and love him was because Brody let her in—a privilege he never granted his wife who woefully knew it and suffered.

* * *

Many men keep their light hidden under a bushel that even a paleontologist could not excavate. A man I know revealed he was looking for the woman he was born to love. I asked, "Do you share your most intimate secrets?" The man quickly jumped, "No! Why share information that can be used against me?" I responded, "That's distrust." The man defended, "That's smart."

This wealthy know-it-all is now 83, he has had a heart attack, he's been divorced three times, he's alone, and depressed. He recently shared, "The only thing that matters is to have a deep love." He never realized that this "deep love" must be two-way, with him as a contributor. Without giving and receiving, love will fail.

Brene Brown asserts, "We cultivate love when we allow our most vulnerable and powerful selves to be seen and known." That requires the ego of false protection to be deflated, followed by emotional nakedness. How many men are willing to shed their façades?

* * *

The men you will meet next have strong Capital "I" power. As I said earlier, you may not agree with all their stands, but the fact that they used their voices demonstrates their unwavering Capital "I" confidence—and they serve to show the world how it's done.

PART V

REAL MEN WHO STAND UP

Could you imagine a world where men are not punished, cancelled, or blocked for speaking their truth—but are instead rewarded? The following Real Men don't protectively act out, hide, or shut down. They were willing to show their vulnerable underbellies and take on the social consequences, whatever they turned out to be.

These Real Men boldly and unabashedly tell their personal truth without sugar coating it. They are proud of their voices and are emotionally free. Nathanial Branden said, "There is no judgment a person can pass that is more significant than the one passed on himself."

Successful people are rejected more than anyone else—because they're out there. Ultimately, they make their rejection and disappointment into the foundation for their success. When we project ourselves as winners, others treat us that way.

The TV series MASH was rejected by more than 32 producers. People told Beethoven all his symphonies were trash. Critics said that "Gone with the Wind" was never going to be a success. A once unknown Brad Pitt spent his savings to fly 6,000 miles to Budapest to see his then fiancée, Jill Schoelen. When he arrived, he discovered she had dumped him for a director. Sylvester Stallone was turned down by over 1000 agents who told him to go home and learn how to talk. So, he wrote his own movie. Everyone rejected that. But he didn't give up. Finally, one company offered to buy it—if he wouldn't star in it! Who's laughing now?

During the great Chicago fire in 1871, many merchants lost their stores. Except for one, they all left Chicago to start over elsewhere. The one who remained said, "On that spot where my former store had been, I will build the world's greatest store..." That man was Marshall Field. He *visualized* his success. Marshall Field's became a huge upscale department store in Chicago, Illinois before Macy's acquired it in 2005.

Author David DeAngelo advises men, "Stop trying to please mommy and take back your b-lls."

* * *

CHAPTER 23

Chris Rock

Responds to The Slap—One Year Later

He had a full year to contemplate the 2022 Oscars Slap, and he made a few comments at various venues during that time, but Chris Rock never fully addressed Smith's brutal attack. In contrast, Will Smith continued making appearances to lukewarm responses.

For its part, the Academy of Motion Picture Arts and Sciences announced a special "crisis team" to avoid similar beatdowns at the March 12, 2023 Oscars. But Rock himself never responded. That is, until he had a standup special on Netflix called "Chris Rock: Selective Outrage."

During this show, the comedian electrified his one-upmanship by calling out his attacker on every count. He glaringly said he's not a victim and no one will see him sitting down and crying with Oprah or Gayle. He discussed how he always admired Smith. Smith's anger wasn't about him. Then, boom, just as this book explained earlier, Rock proclaimed the attack was caused by Smith's wife's "entanglement" with another man. Rock screamed, "She hurt him way more than he hurt me." Rock's mic-drop was the exclamation point to his finale.

The once-silent-on-this-topic Chris Rock enunciated his power, owned the stage, and took charge. He gave new meaning to "manning-up." He did it eloquently and humorously, not with fists, but with powerful words.

Sun Tzu advises that a leader should strategize to exploit his opponent's weakness (That night, Chris Rock owned the mic!) and win without fighting. During her divorce from her cheating husband, Ivana Trump asserted, "Don't get mad; get everything." It might have taken him a year, but that night Chris Rock did indeed get *everything!*

Rock's standup was the most-streamed comedy special in a measurement week. It jumped to 798 million viewing minutes, making it Number 9 on Nielsen's streaming charts for that week. And it was the classiest revenge performance in television history!

CHAPTER 24

Saifullah Khan

Sues to Reclaim Life after Rape Acquittal

Former Yale student Saifullah Khan, 30, was acquitted of rape in 2018. Yet, he was ousted from the Ivy League institution. He had a $110 million defamation suit pending against the school since 2019. He also fought to bring his accuser, a fellow student, into the suit over the 2018 university hearing that had been conducted shabbily. The Connecticut Supreme Court finally ruled he has the right to sue his accuser for defamation over her statements. The world waits to see the results. Kahn exemplifies a millennial man who refuses to accept the unjustified sullying of his reputation.

CHAPTER 25

Sylvester Stallone

Refuses Bud Light's $100 Million Endorsement Deal

As described earlier, Stallone had a difficult time breaking into the entertainment industry. It was one rejection after another before his career finally took off. Today, after years of great success despite the critics, he got to croon Johnny Paycheck's country song, "Take this job and shove it!" when asked to endorse Bud Light.

He's on this list of Real Men Who Stand Up because Hollywood is fueled by money and power—and the size of this offer was enormous. But after being shot down so many times at the start of his career, the man stood by his hard-earned principles. Whether you agree with his stand or not, how many people in Stallone's smoke-and-mirrors industry would have done the same?

CHAPTER 26

Greg O'Brien

Videos His Demeaning Fight against Alzheimer's

Greg was an attractive, successful award-winning investigative reporter in total command of eloquent thoughts and language. Then, without warning, the 59-year-old was diagnosed with Alzheimer's.

In the gripping documentary, "Have You Heard about Greg?" journalist O'Brien, put this "shhh-don't-tell-anyone" illness front and center. With raw transparency, he recorded without embarrassment how he was confronting his 24/7 struggles against the body that had turned on him. His goal was for people to understand this disease and fight to irradicate it.

Unlike other men, Greg shamelessly invited the world to experience his inappropriate behaviors, his rage, his loss of self-control, his plummeting self-esteem, his family's depressions and frustrations, his impending bankruptcy from medical bills, and his two attempted suicides. All on video. Greg's honest story is raw and unfiltered.

Most people live life unconsciously, mindlessly taking one step after another. But Greg said he was deliberately honoring his (and my) favorite philosopher:

Sun Tzu
"Tactics without strategy is the noise before defeat."

Written from the scope of a true investigative reporter, as his body deteriorated, Greg chose the strategy of not treating his accompanying cancers. He titles this last act his "Exit Strategy." O'Brien will leave this world having bravely exposed a dent on a killer disease. For men who won't even wear a nickel-sized blood sugar monitor on their arm, this journalist provides a worthy role model.

CHAPTER 27

Johnny Depp

Defeats Ex-Wife in Defamation Suit

    This renowned actor chose to bare his personal struggles with drugs and alcohol just to overturn his ex-wife's defaming of him as a "domestic abuser." In 2010, The Guinness Book of World Records named Johnny Depp the world's highest-paid actor, with earnings of $75 million.

    Depp's marriage to actress Amber Heard lasted from 2015 to 2017. They met on the set of "The Rum Diary" in 2011. When actors fall in love while working together, they know each other between little else than "action" and "cut." But they don't know each other in daily life.

    Heard alleged that Depp had been verbally and physically abusive throughout their relationship. In 2018, Heard wrote an op-ed piece in the Washington Post in which she described herself as "a public figure representing domestic abuse." Although she never mentioned her ex-husband's name,

Depp's lawyers argued that his reputation and his future re-hiring by Disney were tainted by her article. He sued her for $50 million.

She countersued him for twice that amount, claiming that his team defamed her by calling her abuse claims a "hoax."

Heard's former private investigator, Paul Barresi, was hired by her in preparation for the trial to prove that Depp was a serial abuser. After interviewing over 100 of Depp's associates, there was no one who would attest to Depp's abuse. But Barresi did say that Heard was one of the "most egregious leeches" there were, and she used Depp to get ahead in Hollywood. She was an opportunist who took advantage of her husband by playing on his fragility spawned by a volatile and violent mother.

Depp won the case. The jury found that all the statements from Heard's op-ed were false, these statements *did* defame her ex-husband, and they were made with "actual malice," a legal requirement imposed upon public officials and public figures when they file libel suits. (The law states that public personas should be held to a higher standard in proving defamation claims.)

Depp said, "Speaking the truth was something that I owed to my children and to all those who have remained steadfast in their support of me. I feel at peace knowing I have finally accomplished that. The jury gave me my life back. I hope my quest to have the truth be told will have helped others, men or women, who have found themselves in my situation."

One side of the political aisle opined that Depp's win would crush the often unscrupulous #MeToo complainers. The other side worried that women will cease speaking out against domestic and sexual violence. Unphased by the political innuendo, consumers continue to flock to stores for Depp's fragrance, Sauvage by Dior!

CHAPTER 28

Dr. Peter McCullough

World Expert on COVID Opposes Government Mandates

Peter McCullough, M.D. is an internist, cardiologist, epidemiologist, and the Chief Scientific Officer of the Wellness Company. He has spent years combating the SARS-CoV-2 virus and has reviewed thousands of reports, and has participated in scientific congresses, group discussions, and press releases. He is considered among the world's experts on COVID-19.

Since the pandemic, McCullough has been decrying the vaccine and its dangers, and saying that early treatment options have been suppressed. The scientific community discredited and shunned him. In 2021, he was sued by Baylor Scott and White Health who alleged he had violated their separation agreement by "claiming he is affiliated" with their institution. The case was dismissed with prejudice, meaning no lawsuit arising from the same set of facts can be filed by the parties again.

McCullough beamed, "This is a strong victory for freedom of speech. My analyses and conclusions have been accurate, consistent, and have always been my own, not those of any institution."

One newspaper commented that the enormous crowd giving McCullough standing ovations during his presentation at the Bartlesville Community Center was testimony to the low 43 percent vaccination rate in Washington County, Oklahoma. One of Oklahoma's top infectious disease physicians, Dr. Anuj Malik, director of infection prevention and control at Ascension St. John, called the rally a "politically motivated, ideological speech by a modern-day quack."

McCullough boldly announced, "This is more than a medical topic. Now our freedom, our jobs, our schools, somehow everything got linked to COVID-19."

A group of Houston nurses hired him as a so-called "expert witness in their appeal against a vaccine mandate at Houston Methodist. The media reported McCullough's claims are largely uncorroborated, one of which being that a person who already had COVID does not need the vaccine, and that it can be harmful to those who already have natural immunity.

An interview with Kat Mische Elle described McCullough's meager beginnings and his self-funding of every car, tuition, dorm payment, and meal he ate. "I knew that I could have everything stripped away from me down to nothing—and I could build myself back up again."

He described his drive to know more than he learned in medical school: "Each day I would tell myself 'I'm going to read another chapter, I'm going to read one or two more after it, then I'm going to take some more notes. After that, I'm going to go back to what I have read and I'm going to ask myself questions to see what I learned. Then I'm going to close the book, and I'm going to get a piece of paper to draw out all the chemical reactions and make sure I got them right. I will double-check those results. This was my regular daily study routine all through school." Who wouldn't want to have this kind of thorough and caring physician treating him?

During COVID he said, "Everything I knew to be true was suddenly very confusing." He fought the establishment over the controversial vaccine's safety and efficacy. To combat his negative press, he built an online presence at The Wellness Company, and I have even purchased his products. McCullough says, "Be bold and relentless. It's the only way to get things done."

CHAPTER 29

Bill Ackman

Shouts What Others Only Whisper: "DEI Is Racist"

Bill Ackman is a hedge fund manager who is founder and CEO of Pershing Square Capital Management. His net worth is estimated at $4 billion. He graduated from Harvard College and earned an MBA from Harvard Business School—and this Real Man dared to talk back.

As a Jewish Harvard alumnus, he was appalled by antisemitic rhetoric and the harassment of Jewish students that emerged after the Hamas attack on Israel on October 7, 2023. He wrote a 5,200 word essay on X that was viewed 36 million times. Ackman raged that 34 Harvard student organizations supported Hamas, "a globally recognized terrorist organization holding Israel 'solely responsible' for Hamas' barbaric and heinous acts." He described how antisemitism "exploded on campus" thanks to DEI, and protestors violated Harvard's code of conduct—while President Claudine Gay stood silent.

As he started doing his research, Ackman found that DEI—Diversity, Equity, and Inclusion—"was not what I had naively thought these words meant." They mean "capitalism is racist, Advanced Placement exams are racist, IQ tests are racist, corporations are racist, or in other words, any merit-based program, system, or organization is racist."

He noted that after George Floyd's death, DEI took off without pushback, because challengers were called "racist," which destroyed jobs and reputations and got people cancelled.

Ackman screamed what others only dared to whisper: "DEI is racist because reverse racism is racism." And racism against whites is as egregious as it is for people with other skin tones. Further, the billionaire Democrat announced that DEI is "inconsistent with basic American values. The E for 'Equity' is currently about equality of *outcome*, not equality of *opportunity*."

"But here we are in 2024, required to use skin color to effect outcomes in admissions (recently deemed illegal by the Supreme Court), in business (likely illegal yet it happens nonetheless) and in government (I also believe in most cases to be illegal, except apparently in government contracting). DEI is a racist and illegal movement." And with that, Bill Ackman started a firestorm.

It was almost 30 years ago when I taught in the South Bronx and was denied a school principal's position by my black interviewer. He kindly admitted to this young, starry-eyed white woman that the school district wanted a Hispanic for the position. I was the only candidate with a Ph.D. and New York State certification as a school principal. But my skin tone was not what they were seeking. Ackman's descriptions are accurate, but this has been occurring for decades, whether or not we put it under the aegis of DEI.

Bill Ackman insists it's not okay to select candidates when they're not qualified—like former black Harvard President Claudine Gay. Her leadership deficits were obvious after October 7, he said. Ackman especially took Harvard's board to task, and cautioned them in their selection of the next school president. He closed his essay asking for well-educated and trained leaders "that will help save us from ourselves."

Because of Ackman's powerful noisemaking, political backlash and legal challenges have been building against DEI programs. Challenging Sherita Golden's missive declaring that all white people, Christians, and men are "privileged," a healthcare watchdog group, "Do No Harm," demanded that Johns Hopkins Medicine eliminate its toxic Diversity, Equity, and Inclusion program. The group disavowed Golden's "empty" apology, and stated, "Johns Hopkins needs to completely eliminate their DEI department and channel those resources toward the primary objective of preparing the next generation of healthcare professionals to give the highest quality care to all patients."

A survey by employment law firm Littler Mendelson PC,

examined DEI practices for employers. They found that so far only one percent of companies reported a decrease in their DEI efforts, even after the Supreme Court's ruling on affirmative action sparked increased scrutiny and lawsuits.

Organizations are now auditing and assessing their initiatives, instead of quickly eliminating them. Social change takes time. Quota systems with some jobs reserved for minority candidates run afoul of the law and could be subject to litigation.

In 2024, Econ Journal Watch published a report that the global consulting firm McKinsey & Company conducted bogus research in 2015, 2018, 2020, and 2023. Their findings were not valid or reliable. McKinsey continued to tout a correlation between Diversity, Equity, and Inclusion (DEI) programs and corporate profits. But the findings cannot support the argument that financial performance will improve with increased racial/ethnic diversity of their executives.

Elaine Donnelly, president of the Center for Military Readiness, said the "Race-conscious DEI policies are making personnel shortages worse." There is now a national security risk based on the bogus findings of McKinsey!

In his book, "The Third Awokening: A 12-Step Plan for Rolling Back Progressive Extremism," Eric Kaufmann discusses the youthquake that has taken over our institutions of higher learning. Especially among young women, sensitivity to minorities is more important than free speech, truth, or merit. Kids won't outgrow wokeness over time. He submits that only by reforming our schools can we avert this civilizational train wreck.

Change is beginning at some companies. Kirsten Fleming writes in the New York Post, "If 2023 was peak woke, 2024 will be known as the year that DEI died—with corporations finally admitting it's all a shakedown by Lefty activists." Finally, Bud Light created a new ad for their original customers as post-DEI damage control. After losing a billion dollars, this is their mea culpa for shedding its brand DNA and core customer base.

In May 2024, the elite Massachusetts Institute of Technology (MIT) tossed its controversial diversity hiring requirement. It was the first influential university to rid DEI. They admitted it simply doesn't work. Ford, John Deere, Zoom, Meta, Loew's, and Google made cuts to their DEI departments or abolished them altogether. The assassination attempt on President Donald Trump spotlighted the Secret Service's goal of increasing the number of female agents, and led to more criticism of DEI. Elon Musk took aim at CrowdStrike's DEI policy after their biggest IT global outage in history.

However, Delta Airlines dropped the "ladies and gentlemen" gate greeting to become a more inclusive company in the name of DEI. Harley-Davidson went woke and alienated those who identified with the motorcycle's muscular masculinity. The argument continues.

In his deep, robust voice, Black Lieutenant Governor of North Carolina, Mark Robinson, exclaimed, "My version of

DEI is Discipline, Excellence, and Intelligence." In support of his requirements for rising to the top is the new Internet meme "Didn't Earn It," which Republican Vice Presidential pick, DJ Vance quoted in a speech.

Then the news broke that gullible Facebook and Nike fell for a scam from their own former diversity program manager, Barbara Furlow-Smiles. Companies will do practically anything not to be labeled "racist "or "white supremist." Smiles played on corporate fears and created fake events from which she was able to scam $5 million. She was sentenced to five years in jail and a demand to repay a large sum.

Meanwhile, the Cornell Free Speech Alliance accused Cornell University of "corrupting" its science, math, and engineering programs by rejecting 21 percent of prospective professors whose views were considered against the school's woke ideology.

Black author Adam B. Coleman opined in the New York Post, "We fall for scams when we become so desperate for an outcome that we're willing to suspend belief and overlook common sense. Ego prevents industry leaders from hearing our warnings about the falsehoods they're being fed."

As the commencement speaker and recipient of "Hero of Israel" award, Democrat Senator John Fetterman told Yeshiva University graduates that he was "profoundly disappointed" in his alma mater, Harvard University, for its unwillingness to address antisemitism. He dramatically whipped off the Harvard academic hood he wore and received a standing ovation.

Still, with all the negative rumblings around DEI, in May 2024, Bill Ackman, now framed as an anti-DEI activist, was confronted by Wall Street bigwigs at a conference devoted to DEI. Executives criticized Ackman for saying that DEI was a racist and illegal movement.

His response to Bloomberg News was, "I have written thousands of words about my nuanced views on this important topic. I would ask that people read them to fully understand my perspective." Without raising his fists or his tone, he chose not to regurgitate his position for those who didn't do their homework. Ackman is a Real Man.

CHAPTER 30

Ted Sarandos

Defends Netflix's Programming No Matter Who Is Offended

In 2021, Dave Chappelle's Netflix special, "The Closer," included jokes about transgender people. Some Netflix employees protested by walking out of their employer's Los Angeles headquarters.

Netflix's co-chief executive officer and chief content officer is Ted Sarandos. To the surprise of cancel culture advocates, Sarandos shockingly didn't cave. Instead, he defended Chappelle: "The only way comedians can figure out where the line is, is by crossing the line once in a while. I think it's very important to the American culture to have free expression."

Sarandos continued, "We're programming for a lot of diverse people who have different opinions and different tastes and different styles, and yet we're not making everything for everybody. We want something for everybody, but everything's not going to be for everybody."

He unabashedly told protesters, "If you find it hard to support our content breadth, Netflix may not be the best place for you."

The conservative Daily Caller celebrated Sarandos's stand with the headline, "Netflix Puts Its Woke Employees On Notice with Blunt Memo."

In 2022, also on Netflix, Ricky Gervais had a special called "SuperNature." He joked about transgender women and the debate around bathroom access. Sarandos said his remarks about Chappelle also applied to Gervais. On the other side of the political aisle, Variety's headline sarcastically retorted, "Ricky Gervais Anti-Trans Special Proves Netflix Is on No One's Side But Its Own."

CHAPTER 31

Dan Crenshaw

Blinded Former Navy Seal Touts "Never Be a Victim"

In 2012, on his third tour of duty in Afghanistan, a roadside bomb took Navy Seal Dan Crenshaw's right eye. After re-learning the gift of sight in his good eye, he rebuffed pity. He concluded that people must meet life's toughest challenges (like surviving combat with bullets flying over your head and working to regain your eyesight) without being a victim.

In his book, "Fortitude: American Resilience in the Era of Outrage," his message is to lighten up, toughen up, and get to work on what's really important.

Crenshaw says our society desperately needs tough love. Like the children's book by Kevin Sorbo, he cautions against seeking safe, cushiony spaces. He advises to navigate life with a sense of humor and the knowledge that whatever anyone else says or does, you and you alone control your destiny.

A Republican congressman from Texas, Crenshaw

announced a bill to slash funding for schools that mandate students to sign Diversity, Equity, and Inclusion (DEI) statements, committing themselves to woke oaths at the expense of the allegedly "privileged." Crenshaw blames DEI as the culprit of a toxic campus culture that sets up oppressor versus oppressed. Colleges and universities should be blocked from compelling students to reveal their "race, color, ethnicity, or national origin." He's another Real Man standing up for what he believes.

CHAPTER 32

Ricky Gervais

Pushes the Oscar Envelope of Controversy

Ricky Gervais is an English comedian, actor, writer, producer, and director. As the host of the 77th Golden Globes awards show in 2020, he did what countless viewers have been saying for years as these shows' ratings have consistently dropped. He told the A-list winners not to get political: "Celebrities are in no position to lecture the public about anything."

"If you do win an award tonight, don't use it as a platform to make a political speech. You know nothing about the real world," the comedian continued.

"Most of you spent less time in school than Greta Thunberg," the 17-year-old climate activist. "So, if you win, come up, accept your little award, thank your agent and your god, and f— off."

Hollywood award shows have become increasingly political, with actors using these platforms to rail on hot-button issues and politicians they dislike, mainly Donald

Trump. Ratings for these awards shows have consistently plummeted, except at the Golden Globes in 2024. So, in 2020, Gervais stood up for his viewers, not his A-list colleagues. This caveat should have been issued years ago, but no one had the guts until this Real Man did.

Despite Gervais' warning, performers who read other people's lines and "know nothing about the real world" continue to press their political agendas. Robert De Niro made a spectacle of himself outside Donald Trump's hush money trial in Manhattan, screaming at a Trump supporter, "You're a f---ing idiot."

The National Association of Broadcasters quickly rescinded a previous invitation to a philanthropy award for the "Raging Bull" star: "While we strongly support the right of every American to exercise free speech and participate in civic engagement, it is clear that Mr. De Niro's recent high-profile activities will create a distraction from the philanthropic work we were hoping to recognize." De Niro got cancelled.

The conversion of a platform set up to award merit is becoming more widespread, even outside the realm of entertainment. A 34-year-old Palestinian American labor and delivery nurse at NYU Langone Health in New York City was awarded for her compassion for moms who grieved their deceased babies. Yet, her acceptance speech accused Israel of committing "genocide" in Gaza—which was her second warning about bringing her personal beliefs into the workplace. She was fired.

In Beverly, Massachusetts, Richard Dreyfuss was asked to speak at The Cabot Theatre about the 1975 movie" Jaws" in which he had starred. But he went off script on the Right side of the aisle and criticized Barbara Streisand, transgender youth, the Academy Awards' inclusivity rules, and gender affirmation. Theatre goers walked out.

Whether a personality is a civilian or a celebrity, whether that person is Right or Left, Gervais's words continue to ring true: stick to what audiences came to hear you discuss.

Now we learn that celebrities are being "shamed" to speak out on various causes during these polarized times. If the voice of an A-lister is especially absent from the media, a new group of online thugs gives them the "digitine "or "digital guillotine."

Digitine has replaced cancel culture. Getting the digitine means you'll be digitally blocked if you *fail* to throw your money and your name behind a hot cause, despite your personal political views. It's A-list blackmail because celebrities' careers and incomes depend on their digital exposure. Blackmailing is illegal. These internet Mafia-style members aim to impact celebs' incomes with the attitude, "We gave them their platform. It's time to take it back."

The digitine already fell on Selena Gomez, Zendaya, Justin Bieber, the Kardashians, and Taylor Swift for failing to show support for Palestinians. Since this scheme is now in the open, I question each political diatribe I hear from an A-lister.

CHAPTER 33

Dr. Jordan Peterson

*Leads the Way for Strong Men,
Loses License and University Credentials*

Psychologist Jordan Peterson, Ph.D. former professor at numerous academic institutions including Harvard, had been writing and lecturing for many years. His following has been described as "cult-like" and his books have sold millions. His anti-woke bestseller is "12 Rules for Life: An Antidote to Chaos."

As he and his platform became more recognizable, Peterson began to speak out about gender issues. In June 2022, Peterson posted a tweet misgendering transgender actor Elliot Page, calling Page's surgeon "a criminal." His Twitter account (before it became X) was suspended upholding the "hateful conduct policy." When Peterson was told to delete the tweet or lose his account, he responded, "I would rather die than do that." YouTube demonetized Peterson's videos, one about his Twitter suspension and another quoting his statement that gender-affirming care was "Nazi medical experiment-level wrong." In November 2022, after Elon Musk took Twitter's reins, Peterson's Twitter account was restored.

The psychologist has been named a "manfluencer" and has been outspoken about an ongoing "crisis of masculinity" in which "the masculine spirit is under assault." He said, "If men are pushed too hard to feminize, they will react with more interest in harsh political ideology."

To Peterson, culture is "symbolically, archetypally, mythically male," while "chaos—the unknown—is symbolically female." Peterson said, "Confused gay kids are being convinced they're transsexual. Well, that's not so good for gay people, is it? There's certainly a lot of confused adolescents who could be enticed into narcissistic abnormality as a consequence of attention-seeking."

He announced that gender-neutral singular pronouns were radical Left ideologies that he detests, and frighteningly similar to Marxism that killed 100 million people in the 20th century. Gender-neutral pronouns have not been universally accepted. A man on an online dating profile warned potential mates, "Automatic demotion if you do that pronoun thing. If I can't tell you're obviously female, it's already a non-starter."

Because Peterson refused to buy into "that pronoun thing," the University of Toronto sent him letters of warning, saying that free speech had to be within the boundaries of human rights legislation. His refusal to use preferred personal pronouns of students and faculty upon request could constitute discrimination.

In January 2017 he returned to teach his psychology class at the university. However, as the trans debate heated up at the start of 2023, the College of Psychologists of Ontario ordered Peterson to undergo social media communication coaching. The psychologist denied any wrongdoing and filed for judicial review. His appeal was reviewed by three judges of an Ontario court who upheld the college's decision. The college ordered Peterson to pay for the costs of his own training and noted that failure to comply could result in the loss of his license in the province. He stood firm on his platform, and his license was revoked.

Writing for the Left-leaning Washington Post, Christine Embe noted that men began donning new identities in 2016. When a confused male university student asked, "What does good masculinity look like?" his male professor admitted he didn't have an answer.

Hearing the buzz about Peterson in 2018, Embe got tickets to a sold-out lecture in Washington D.C. He had achieved rock star status with his fame, notoriety, and millions of book sales. Embe describes him as one of "many Right aligned masculinity gurus" who fill the void in explaining manhood.

She went to the lecture as a skeptic, but left understanding his appeal. Through his display of empathy for young men, the writer saw how he validates their struggles. He tells them they matter, and he excuses their behaviors because "school is tailored to girls." He concurs that being a man today is tough!

Embe writes, "For young men . . . the assumption of a world built to serve them doesn't align with their lived experience, where girls out-achieve them from pre-K to post-graduate studies and 'men are trash' is an acceptable joke." A therapist testified that she observed how Peterson turned a boy into a responsible and successful wage-earning man.

The former non-believer said the curriculum for "Peterson The Savior" highlights positive traits like protectiveness, leadership, and emotional stability. The message is that being masculine is honorable and desirable: "And the fact he's willing to define it outright feels bravely countercultural." This writer from the "other side" nailed the need as well as the cure in this one man.

Like Embe, I attended one of Peterson's large gatherings in a 5,000-seat arena in Phoenix, Arizona. The crowd consisted mostly of young and middle-aged men, with a smattering of women. He explained that he had been cancelled by his university—so he "returned the favor" and built his own online academy! I have since enrolled to learn enlightening information from different masters in their disciplines, information I will not find elsewhere.

I was entranced by Peterson's genuine interest in each audience member's question. He tossed his head back, closed his eyes, and carefully *heard, digested, and responded to* each heartfelt plea for guidance. He was genius, and I was blown away!

Peterson feels he was cancelled from truth, love, and relationships. His philosophy is, "When you're called upon to speak, take the risk and speak up."

With a VIP ticket, I got to converse with him for a few minutes. I told him about this book, "Real Men Don't Go Woke," and said he's in it as one of my "Real Men." He asked that I send him a copy after it's published, and we exchanged contact information. When I posted our photo together, my social media followers commented how lucky I was to have conversed with this giant. I agree!

CHAPTER 34

Kevin Sorbo

Exits Hollywood's Woke Agenda that Mocks Men

I spoke with Kevin Sorbo at a meeting of New York Media Initiative (nee MasterMedia). He was still living in Los Angeles and becoming more unhappy with his industry and its politics. You've read about him earlier in this book. The man who played Hercules began to post his views on social media and he kept getting cancelled. Who cancels mighty Hercules? He left California for Florida. He is on this list of Real Men Who Stand Up because despite Hollywood's cold shoulder, he continues to speak his mind by making family-positive movies. Nothing will keep Hercules down.

CHAPTER 35

Jon Stewart

*Quits Apple TV Show when
He's Refused Creative Control*

On Apple TV+, Democrat actor-comedian Jon Stewart had been doing his "The Problem With Jon Stewart" show for two years. By the second year, some viral episodes led to an Emmy nomination for outstanding talk series. Apple demanded final say over the show's content, concerned that Stewart would hit sensitive topics regarding China and AI. Apple is one of a few American tech companies that have a presence in China, and Apple products rely on components for their iPhone, iPad, and AirPods made in that country.

Some American entertainment companies are careful not to upset their relationship with China, fearing financial repercussions. China has already punished Warner Bros. Discovery, the National Basketball Association, and the Walt Disney Company because employees spoke badly about the

Chinese government. So, Apple tries to protect the delicate balance to preserve its economic clout.

Many show hosts would have caved to the pressure to keep their show on the air. But Stewart refused to be held down by Apple's constraints, and instead chose to walk.

I know firsthand about the thrust of a powerful TV network's wishes against your own. I have had red hair from the day I was born. Over the years, it has provided me with a recognizable trademark. In the 1980s and 1990s, I appeared on every show from Howard Stern to Dateline to daytime talk to nighttime news. One show on which I spent years appearing was "Sally Jessy Raphael" on NBC. I had a huge following and fan mail from countries around the world.

One day, Sally's producers summoned me to their office. They requested that I alter my hair color. I was shocked. They said that Sally had cut her hair to my trendy short style, and now she also dyed it red. They said that when Sally and I had our backs to the audience, people could not distinguish us. Now they wanted me to dye my hair to another color. Sally and I were not the same height or girth, and it felt like the producers were asking me to cut off a limb.

I told them I've never had another hair color, and I won't change it now. They threatened to fire me if I didn't comply. I imagined my TV career going up in smoke. But I stood my ground and didn't change the color of my hair. I remained on the show until bogus rumors circulated that I was going to replace Sally with a show of my own. Although that was not true, Sally saw me as competition—which was probably what was behind her desire to cut and dye her hair to look like mine. She kicked me off her show. A few months later, Twentieth Century Fox taped a TV pilot for the Dr. Gilda show, totally independent of Sally's show.

Only a handful of people in the world get to have their own nationally syndicated TV show. The opportunity was a gift from heaven, especially because I didn't even have an agent or entertainment attorney. But audiences trusted me and Hollywood decision-makers called me "mediagenic."

Schadenfreude is rampant in an industry whose stakes are very high. Badmouthing and nasty comments got back to me from people I thought were my allies. I continued to stand strong despite the nastiness. The Hollywood mogul in charge loved the "Dr. Gilda" show pilot and wanted to get it on the air at once. Sadly, he suffered an untimely death. Fox dropped all his proposed shows, including mine.

There is always a reason for things that happen or don't, but I didn't get to discover what that was at the time. I did, years later . . .

<u>Gilda-Gram</u>
Each rejection is God's protection.

Television taught me how strong I am in my determination to maintain my identity, my values, and my backbone—despite potential career-shattering consequences. It taught me that if people are *not* talking about me in such a public arena, something is wrong. I look in the mirror today with fiercer eyes and the determination it has taken to even write this book.

I never met Jon Stewart, but I identify with his stand to maintain his dignity for what he believed was right. He's now doing another show, and he's killing it. Good for him!

CHAPTER 36

Unknown Man

*Confronts Abusive Ex and Kids
—to Internet Applause!*

The headline on the app TooFab, a subsidiary of Fox Corporation, read, "Dad Gets Overwhelming Support For Telling Kids He Doesn't Give a Sh-t If Their Sick Mom Dies, Doesn't Love Them."

It sounds heartless. An uncertain 56-year-old Unknown Man posted a letter to an anonymous forum because he wondered if he had been too harsh with his kids, and he asked a Reddit "AITA ("Am I The Asshole?") question.

When Unknown Man was 37 years old, he was diagnosed with pancreatic cancer. Although the disease was found early, the man was not expected to survive. A month after the diagnosis, his wife left him, took his kids aged 14, 12, and 11, the house, and their savings. His wife's excuse was that she didn't want to be his nurse as she watched him die. As an only child whose parents died in his 20s, he had no other family to give him support during his terrifying demise.

The doctors removed the tumor and administered chemo. Miraculously, the pancreatic cancer went into remission, which is unusual for that disease. The man tried to be involved in his kids' lives, but his ex-wife remarried eleven months after the remission, and Unknown Man felt replaced. Despite volunteering to pay child support in exchange for his ex's promise not to deplete his savings entirely, he continued to reach out, send birthday and holiday gifts, and make phone calls to his kids—but he got back monosyllabic responses or none at all. Eventually, he gave up. He fought for the kids until the youngest was 22. He said that experience hurt him almost as much as the cancer.

He married a co-worker, and they parented two children. He wrote, "It still hurts, but I love my new family, and they actually give a sh-t about me."

Fast forward to two decades later. Unknown Man's ex-wife was diagnosed with terminal heart disease and the family was struggling financially. For the first time in ten years, his children called and asked their father to lunch. He didn't want to go, but his current wife convinced him to see them because it seemed they were offering an olive branch.

When they all gathered, the kids didn't ask how the man had been doing all these years. They jumped right in and requested financial support for the medical bills for their mom. They pleaded that even if he didn't love her, he should contribute for the sake of his children.

Unknown Man asked them with whom they had spent the last two decades of Father's Day. He asked why he should care about a woman who took everything from him and left him alone to face death. Why should he worry about the kids who wouldn't even see him before his surgery or at any point when he was dying? They sat silent. He continued, "I don't care how bad her dying hurts you guys because I care about you as much as you care about me—not in the slightest. I won't help because I don't love her or you guys." He got up from the table and left.

He asked the forum, "AITA?"

Besides a few bleeding hearts who called his actions coldblooded, the rest of the Internet overwhelmingly supported Unknown Man and said he was absolutely right. Like it or not, this is what the art of re-taking your power looks like. And people who had enough of the one-sided and biased-against-men support system applauded the outcome.

I know men who still jockey for a position in the lives of children who have discarded them. Most of these men are over 50. One man of 73 described how he still keeps an open calendar should his estranged son choose to reach out. Although he's no longer in contact with his ex-wife, when the man had a recent health scare, he shared the bad news with his progeny. He never heard back. *Ouch!*

CHAPTER 37

YOU

*If You Haven't Yet Claimed Your Voice,
the Time is Now!*

It takes tremendous courage to stand alone with your convictions, knowing you might be the last man standing, and knowing you have little support.

- When were you asked to compromise your values for something you did not believe in?
- When did you decide to take an unpopular stand?
- How did you reach your resolve to be the odd man out?
- What consequences did you experience?
- If time has passed, would you now say it was worth it?

There are so many more Real Men I could have added to this list if not for space restrictions. Like the courageous Elon Musk for continuing to stand up for what he feels is right instead of what is politically popular. Like and the entire cast and crew of "Sound of Freedom" that fought against Hollywood when it refused to produce or distribute the child-trafficking movie. Like Arizona's Sheriff Mark Lamb whose son, son's fiancé, and baby were killed by a drunk driver, yet who still ran for U.S. Senate to clean up the country's southern border. The Sheriff lost the primary to Kari Lake, but nonetheless, in the classiest way, he videotaped a support speech for her. Like Mohit Ramchandani, the writer and director of "City of Dreams," a film about human trafficking, already being denigrated for speaking out about these atrocities. Like lots of other men unnamed here who raise their voices above the deafening woke opposition.

In a world that catcalls heterosexual men "weak" and "feckless," these men refuse to go down without defending their platforms. I salute them!

I am compiling a list from my readers and followers for my website. Please nominate A Real Man (someone you know or someone in the news) on the form at www.DrGilda.com. Let's keep building this list.

The more men we can gather, the stronger and healthier the role models we can build for our children.

* * *

CONCLUSION

Every Setback Re-Sets Us for a Better Path

Creating a strong YOU leaves a vacant position for a person who conforms. Observe how that conformist is floundering and how he needs direction and support to stop his internal war!

<u>Sun Tzu</u>
"All warfare is based on deception."

Do we want a deceit-filled life where every word is guarded, and all uniqueness is squashed? Neither love nor success can exist without free-flowing trust. We've been traveling down this rabbit hole for too long, and we must quell this now, because

<u>Sun Tzu</u>
"A kingdom that has once been destroyed can never come again into being . . ."

Therefore,

<u>Sun Tzu</u>
"In peace, prepare for war,
in war prepare for peace."

Our interpersonal communications must become transparent now. Why waste miserable years wondering when you will feel safe before you tell your story to someone you trust?

A 2008 romantic comedy, "The Women," adapted from the Clare Boothe Luce 1937 play, depicted a wealthy suburban housewife doing her chores and charities while Hedge-Fund-Hubby bonked a sexy sidepiece. After the usual crying and chaos, the housewife found her purpose and rekindled the passions she had put on the back burner for the sake of married life. She became an accomplished dress designer, and, of course, once Hubby glimpsed her starring role, he wanted her back. He sent flowers with a note that would stop any woman in her tracks: "I want to get to know you again. Have I missed my chance?"

With her newfound strength, she responded, "I'm gonna own up to my part in this. How could I share myself with you *if I had no idea who I was?*"

Similarly, if a man doesn't know who he is, he won't know what he values or what he's looking for. When self-sufficiency and self-care are absent, a relationship with *anyone* will fail.

The former housewife-turned-designer said, "I want things now that I put aside and I'm gonna get them. And anybody who is part of my life is gonna want those things for me. But this is gonna be hard. This is hard, hard work. It doesn't happen overnight. And if you can accept all of that, I will see you Tuesday at 8. That's all I have available. I'm a very busy person."

The voiceless person the housewife used to be became proud of the strong woman she had become. And in this movieland fantasy, her husband was newly fascinated by her and wanted to be part of the life of his exciting and independent wife. When we throw a pebble in the ocean, there's a rippling effect. All relationships depend on each of us to play fair, and that will affect and infect each other. One person can't do it alone.

Men, acknowledge your dreams. Manifest your Capital "I." Before you seek a mate, proudly announce, "I am loving my life—and I have something to contribute to yours."

This awareness came to the former "Dr. Quinn, Medicine Woman" actress Jane Seymour at 72, with four past marriages and four children. She said that in all her former relationships, she neglected putting herself first. She's now partnered with a robust 73-year-old man, and she says that sex is built on their *emotional intimacy*. Before she found him, she had pursued who she was *alone*. Now, because she knows herself and her body, she says, "I feel like I'm both experienced and 16 years old. I truly feel sex and intimacy is better at my age than it ever was before."

Not everyone is willing to be alone to figure things out.

While doing my radio show in New York, a man called in to say he had just divorced his wife, and he was miserable and lonely. He asked where he could meet women. I told him not to meet anyone until he understood the basis of his breakup. He screamed into the airwaves, "Hey, Doc! Are you saying I should put myself on ice?" I responded, "Unless you determine what happened and why, I promise you'll repeat the same pattern in the future with your next woman. And you'll experience heartache again. Determine who you are before you give yourself to someone new." He hung up on me.

Our culture has had it backwards; it's pushed us towards relationship without first knowing solo-ship. Once men feel good about themselves, they can feel safe to show their vulnerabilities and share their dreams.

The inner bickering between "woke "and" toxic" has made men fearful of being heard. So, they suppress and hide through the 10 camouflages I listed above to protect themselves. Women play a role in men's demise. Women must know exactly who they are and what they want.

Farrell notes that our culture has never accepted male vulnerability. This requires women to listen differently to men, but it also requires men to courageously speak their truth even if it means being ostracized, which may feel dangerous at first.

Women must make it safe for men to share their underbelly. They should make their guy feel wanted and needed. Hear his anger, but peel it away to feel his vulnerability. And then give him space to exit confusion and vocalize his manly concerns without being his critical mother.

I love Maher's analogy that "masculinity is coffee: even when you decaffeinate it, there's still a little caffeine in there." In the same way, a Real Man may occasionally be a bit "toxic" and a bit "woke." As long as his core is genuine, so what? He'll know he has a voice in a safe woman's presence, and he will not fear using it. Secure women will cut him some slack, work through his issues with him, and accept him for all he is. He will offer the same kindness to her. Neither gender has a perfected model, and it is our many layers that give us our variegated substance.

Bill Maher's decaf analogy can only exist and thrive when respect for self and others is part of the equation. The artificial protective barriers I enumerate here must be de-constructed. The hiding mechanisms must cease. Once a man is unencumbered in his light, he'll comfortably find that surviving is nowhere near the wonder of thriving.

So, how do you take your coffee?

Love, because that's all that matters,

—Dr. Gilda

SOURCES FOR EXPANSION

Written & Audio Works

- Abraham Maslow, "A Theory of Human Motivation," 2020 public domain (audio)

- Avrum Weiss, "Hidden in Plain Sight: How Men's Fears of Women Shape their Intimate Relationships," 2021, excerpted in "Psychology Today"

- Bari Weiss, TED Talk, "Courage, the Most Important Virtue" 2024 + The Free Press, www.thefp.com

- Brene Brown, "The Power of Vulnerability: Teachings of Authenticity, Connection, and Courage," 2012; "Men, Women and Worthiness: The Experience of Shame and the Power of Being Enough," 2012

- Bill Maher, "What This Comedian Said Will Shock You," 2024

- Caitlin Roper, "Sex Dolls, Robots and Woman Hating: The Case for Resistance," 2022

- Carolyn Myss, "Why People Don't Heal and How They Can," 1998

- Christiane Northrup, "Women's Bodies, Women's Wisdom (Revised Edition): Creating Physical and Emotional Health and Healing," 2010

- Collette Dowling, "The Cinderella Complex: Women's Hidden Fear of Independence," 1981

- Dan Crenshaw, "Fortitude: American Resilience in the Era of Outrage," 2020

- Daniel Amen, "Change Your Brain, Change Your Life (Revised and Expanded): The Breakthrough Program for Conquering Anxiety, Depression, Obsessiveness, Lack of Focus, Anger, and Memory Problems," 2015

- Daniel Goleman, "Emotional Intelligence," 2005

- Edmond Rostand, "Cyrano de Bergerac," 2012

- Edwin Arlington Robinson, "Richard Cory," poem, 1897

- Elisabeth Kubler Ross, "On Death and Dying," 2014

- Eric Kaufmann, "The Third Awokening: A 12-point Plan for Rolling Back Progressive Extremism," 2024

- Gilda Carle, "Don't Bet on the Prince!" 2011

- Geert Hofstede, "Cultures and Organizations: Software of the Mind, Third Edition," 2010
- Greg Gutfeld, "The King of Late Night," 2023 (Audio)
- Hailey Magee, "Stop People Pleasing and Find Your Power," 2024
- Hale Dwoskin, "The Sedona Method," 2003
- Hugh Prather, "Notes to Myself: My Struggle to Become a person," 1983
- Jim Morrison, "The Collected Works of Jim Morrison: Poetry, Journals, Transcripts, and Lyrics," (Collected in collaboration with Jim Morrison's Estate), 2021
- Jon Clifton (CEO of Gallop), "Blind Spot: The Global Rise of Unhappiness and How Leaders Missed It," 2022
- Jordan Peterson, "12 Rules for Life: An Antidote to Chaos," 2018 + www.petersonacademy.com
- Kevin Sorbo, "The Test of Lionhood," 2023
- Loral Langemeier, "The Millionaire Maker: Act, Think, and Make Money the Way the Wealthy Do," 2006
- M. Curtis McCoy, "How To Be Successful: Think Like A Leader," 2020
- Mark Driscoll, "Act Like a Man: 9 Ways to Punch Life in the Mouth, 2024 + Pastor, Trinity Church, Scottsdale, AZ

- Nathaniel Branden, "The Six Pillars of Self-Esteem: The Definitive Work on Self-Esteem by the Leading Pioneer in the Field," 1995

- Nicholas Eberstadt, "Men without Work: Post-Pandemic Edition (New Threats to Freedom Series), 2022

- Niobe Way, "Rebels with a Cause: Reimagining Boys, Ourselves, and Our Culture" 2024

- Peter McCullough and John Leake, "The Courage to Face COVID-19: Preventing Hospitalization and Death While Battling the Bio-Pharmaceutical Complex," 2022 + The Wellness Company, www.twc.health

- Phillip C. McGraw, "We've Got Issues: How You Can Stand Strong for America's Soul and Sanity," 2024 + Merit Street Media, www.meritstreetmedia.com

- Prince Harry The Duke of Sussex, "Spare," 2023

- Richard Reeves, "Of Boys and Men," 2024

- Robert Bly, "Iron John: A Book about Men," 2015

- Shannon Ashley, "What Can We Do with All These Broken Woke Men?" 2020

- Sun Tzu, "The Art of War," 2018

- W. Somerset Maugham (1874 – 1945), "The Magician: "It's a very funny thing about life; if you refuse to accept anything but the best, you very often get it," 2014

- Warren Farrell, "The Boy Crisis: Why Our Boys Are Struggling and What We Can Do about It," 2019; "Women Can't Hear What Men Don't Say," 2000 + 6-part lecture series on Peterson Academy, www.PetersonAcademy.com

Movies, Documentaries

- "Broadcast News," 1987
- "Have You Heard about Greg? A Journey through Alzheimer's," 2023, PBS
- "Homeland" series, Showtime, 2011 - 2020
- "Jealousy of Stripping | 50 Ways to Leave Your Lover," Investigation Discovery, YouTube, 2013
- "Not Easily Broken," 2009
- "The Women," 2008
- "The Women—It's All About Men," 1937
- "What the Bleep Do We Know?" 2004 movie
- "Why Movies Need Masculinity," 2022 documentary, YouTube
- "Yellowstone," American neo-Western drama television series, 2018 - 2024
- "15 Minutes of Shame," 2021 documentary, HBO-Max

Music

- Jana Kramer, "I Got the Boy, She Got the Man"
- Blake Shelton, "She Wouldn't Be Gone"
- Brandon Davis, "Tough"
- Johnny Paycheck, "Take This Job and Shove It"
- LeAnn Rimes, "Give"

Made in the USA
Middletown, DE
23 September 2025